WHOLLY
aligned

WHOLLY
alive

Awakening your inner physician

CIARA JEAN ROBERTS

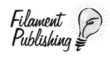

Published by
Filament Publishing Ltd
16, Croydon Road, Waddon, Croydon,
Surrey, CR0 4PA, United Kingdom
Telephone +44 (0)20 8688 2598
Fax +44 (0)20 7183 7186
info@filamentpublishing.com
www.filamentpublishing.com

ISBN 978-1-912635-96-2

Printed by IngramSpark

Disclaimer:
This book is written from my heart and memory bank - as such it is from my own
personal perspective and is not intended to offend any other human. In addition, whilst
I am an experienced therapist working with the modalities of both yoga and nutrition,
my choices are my own when it comes to my health and are not meant as an
encouragement for others to emulate. Part of awakening your inner physician is that it is
your unique journey to discover the medicine for you at any given time, based on
a combination of intuition, knowledge and medical advice.

For my dear Marley — thank you for all your unconditional love, wisdom and support.

Acknowledgements

The birthing of a book is an often solitary journey that requires commitment, ongoing passion on your subject matter and strong self motivation, especially when the old procrastination comes up - and my, it does!

My acknowledgements are in direct relation to this book, so no-one needs to feel excluded; it is not a lifelong list of thank yous - it's for the book project only!

Thank you to my dear friend Dana, who first planted the seed quite some years ago when she asked, 'Ciarita, when are you going to write a book about all of this?'

Thank you to my first editor Parul MacDonald at Cornerstones, who provided such useful advice at the outset on how to tell and craft a story and to always keep the reader in mind. Your final gem of advice that still rings in my ears is, 'Don't give up.'

Thank you to my business coach, Darieth Chisholm, who kept me accountable and was instrumental to me getting the manuscript submitted and keeping the finish line in sight.

Thank you to Katie Rose - my first writing buddy where we scheduled time together to sit down and map out our books. I look forward to yours completing too, Katie!

Thank you to Filamant Publishing. The publishing process can feel opaque and all very new to a first time writer. I feel that through Filament, I have grown my knowledge around the whole process hugely, and am equipped to navigate it for book two! To that end, thank you Sarah Cross for your skilful editing on the entire manuscript to help with flow and chronology. Thank you Clare Clarke for the super typesetting and design.

Thank you to Chris Watson for his humanity and skill.

Thank you to a dear friend Julia Pilkington who asked to read my first chapter, and gave such massively helpful feedback that changed the layout and tone of the first three chapters you now see. Julia, your support and interest is so appreciated.

Thank you to dear Marley for her constant interest and encouragement in my writing progression. It is a gift to allow yourself to be truly seen by your loved ones.

Thank you to my ally, mirror and best friend Anna, who has understood my mission and given me the space I have needed to write, alongside the support I have needed as a human - what an adventure and treasure chest our friendship is. Here's to many more laughs, heartfelt sharing and exciting trips.

Finally, thank you to Bageriat, the tiniest and loveliest Swedish bakery in Covent Garden and to Blackbird Bakery in Crystal Palace - much of this book was birthed in these two places and, as such, I will always hold them dear.

About the author

Ciara Jean Roberts is a yoga teacher and nutritional therapist with a previous credit risk background in private banking. She loves variety! *Wholly Aligned,Wholly Alive*, is her first book and follows the successful publication of a number of articles across media such as *Journal of Kidney Care*, *Yoga Magazine* and *Elephant Journal*. She considers her kidneys amongst her wisest teachers. She lives in vibrant Crystal Palace, London, right next to a wood that she can often be found skipping through.

For fortnightly updates on inspiring, hopeful and helpful content, please sign up to the newsletter via www.whollyaligned.com

For those keen to explore more around how to awaken your inner physician, do listen to the free masterclass, created just for you also available at www.whollyaligned.com

Do also join Ciara on Twitter and Instagram:

@WhollyAligned
#whollyaligned

Contents

Chapter One
The childhood years   9

Chapter Two
Along comes Kenny Kidney   25

Chapter Three
A reorientation   41

Chapter Four
Powerful tools: Nutrition   53

Chapter Five
Powerful tools: Yoga and Shamanic Wisdom   77

Chapter Six
Your wellbeing fund   101

Chapter Seven
The power of the therapeutic rapport   119

Chapter Eight
Finding joy in your recovery   165

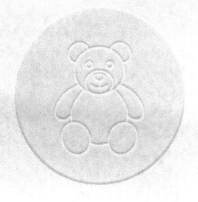

CHAPTER ONE

The childhood years

Born in a land of paradox – apartheid was still the law – I came into the world, into this lifetime, under the glow of the African sun in Johannesburg. In the glorious sunshine in nearby Zambia, where we had moved to from Ireland when I was four years old, we enjoyed our own plentiful garden full of goodness – a vegetable patch, an avocado tree, a pau-pau tree, banana and peach trees. This was a blessed childhood for me.

Life brings us what we need.

Luckily for me, my earlier childhood created very powerful foundations for my journey to come. Strong seeds were planted during that time, which would influence me hugely into adulthood and how, in my own way, I awakened my inner physician.

Upon reflection, I realise now that I had two childhoods. One where I was carefree under the African sun, and the other where I was in a much harsher setting: boarding school in Ireland and then living with an aunt in England. Although it was only a period of two years, in many ways they were very bleak times, and a 180 degree turn away from the warmth of my parents, wholesome food and the Zambia of my earlier years. This was combined with the wider aspect of growing through childhood, as we become more aware of ourselves and more exposed to the actions of the world. Who we are at four is typically far freer than who we are at ten.

I flourished growing up in Zambia. Flourish means to grow luxuriantly, to thrive, and that I did. This was despite a kidney condition that had been diagnosed as a form of glomerular nephritis when I was four years old, following an occurrence of a strep throat bacterial infection. This seemed incidental to me and only required occasional visits to a lovely South African doctor called Professor Thompson, in Johannesburg. I remember the professor having a shock of glorious white hair and kind eyes. Two or three times a year, I would travel with Marley (as I called my mother) and we would combine it with a trip to our close family friends living in the city. So it was all an enjoyable experience with my mother, and I felt completely safe.

In Zambia I felt safe, loved, warm, happy and most definitely healthy. Life was simple and full of music, friends, wellness, innocence, wilderness and vitality. My father was a self-trained musician alongside his profession of accountancy, and played the guitar and mandolin in a lively ceilidh band. This gave me an early insight into the joy and power of creating one's own music and my parents encouraged me to embrace things that I enjoyed, and to really experience life.

Being sent away to boarding school in Dublin at the age of ten, to join my older sister, Aisling, who had already been there a few years, was a shock to my system on many levels. The medical approach in Ireland was far different to South Africa and I no longer enjoyed the experience or, indeed, felt safe. Alongside poor advice to drink processed energy milkshakes daily, being far away from the nature and bounty of Zambia and eating school food, I don't recall my one year at boarding school fondly. I missed my parents hugely and ached for the familiarity of Zambia. I never truly felt at home during my year in Dublin. The weather was colder, the atmosphere bleaker, and I was with a bunch of mixed aged girls, most of whom were away from their own home. I used to get headaches and carried a sense of disconnectedness with me.

And it was here I became very ill. I became less interested in food, started to get fluid retention and more headaches and fatigue, which were indicating a worsening of the kidney condition. It resulted in me having to go to hospital in Dublin. An experience I had to navigate at ten years old, with no trusted adult by my side.

Whilst on the ward in the Dublin hospital, I took a call from Marley, ringing from Zambia. There were no mobile phones at that point, so I sat alone in one of the nurse's or doctor's offices to take the call. She said she would get a flight to come over to Ireland. But I said it was fine, I felt it was a long way to travel and I'd be home soon. This felt like an appropriate reassurance. However, I felt really quite alone and a sense of sadness perfused my system. I had no-one to talk with about how I was feeling, or someone I loved to hold me close. At four years my senior, this was not for my fourteen-year-old sister to take on, although her visits did bring me real comfort. When she visited with her school friend and their parents, her friend brought me a selection of Sweet Valley High books, which I thought was brilliant. I felt very grown up having these teenage books to read.

One incident really brought home to me how alone I was. I was recovering in bed after a kidney biopsy, when one of the nurses came to collect a urine sample with a bed pan. It felt so cold under me that I froze into myself, embarrassed and unable to pee. Sensing this, the nurse turned on the tap and left me in peace for a few moments, after which I easily passed urine. I think I recall this so clearly because it was so telling of how coldly clinical an experience can be for a young child, who has no warmth to lean into.

I left boarding school after the hospitalisation episode and was sent to live with my aunt in Dorset, and attend the same convent school as my cousin. I had mixed feelings about this. I felt excited to start at a new school where my cousin was already settled, yet I still yearned to be at home in Zambia with the safety of my parents, healthy food and a simple life. However, I didn't feel I was able to vocalise these feelings while all the steps were being taken to organise the move. It is only much more recently that I understood the rationale was to keep me in the western medical system. I always had thought it was to prioritise my education. Marley had said she was keen to bring me back to Zambia and put me into the International School in Lusaka. However, my father - Parley - had thought it best to keep me in Europe. Surely this speaks to the inevitable push/pull that goes on in any marriage, especially when it comes to the care of a child. I know this was all with the best of intentions, but it came at such a price to me. It created deep seated feelings of abandonment that I only started to feel into and explore years later, when I was in my thirties.

My care was transferred from Dublin to the U.K and another onslaught of poor advice: this time to drink Hycal, essentially a syrup drink, to keep calorie consumption up. For anyone that understands the body well, loading refined sugar into it is one of the worst things you can do. It adds to inflammation and puts pressure on the kidneys and the endocrine system. This memory still triggers feelings of upset and frustration in me at the complete lack of understanding, and damaging standard protocol. I was not underweight, was normal height for a girl my age and had a regular appetite – so this drink was both unnecessary and harmful. In addition, my aunt did not feed me well, nor understand why I should not be drinking the Hycal, and was watching that I did. She gave me processed foods I had never been given before, such as a white bread roll with cheese and a packet of frazzles for lunch, along with processed cereals for breakfast. It did not feel natural to me to eat this way. This was not the only reason that living with my aunt was deeply distressing. She also had psychological issues which made it really quite an unpleasant year. I was even more unhappy than when at boarding school. That said, I did love the school I was attending. I still returned home to Lusaka for the holidays, but recall being so upset on one flight back to England to return to school that I was physically sick on the plane. I wept to my parents and was desperate to ask them to hold me close and not send me away again. It was so unbearable to be away from them. Feelings that I was unsafe grew deeper and a pervasive mistrust of the medical system was settling into my tissues. I also believed that talking about how I was feeling was futile, and didn't even know how I would without breaking in two.

Thankfully, I was only with this aunt for one academic year and I like to think I had only limited amounts of the Hycal, as it felt so wrong in my body. It speaks to the importance of having a trusted guardian with you as a child, so you feel safe and supported. A doctor cannot assume the adult present is the best fit for the child.

Thankfully, my parents made the decision to leave Zambia for various reasons and come to live in Dorset. This meant I could continue at the school I was at, which I did enjoy and where I had made good friends. It was a relief on many levels, although I felt very sad to be leaving my beloved Africa, which had kept me so well in my younger years.

I wasn't feeling great, however, and still had to be regularly monitored for kidney function. Starting to move through early puberty puts more pressure on one's body, especially if there is an underlying illness. The wheels were turning toward big changes. When I had just turned fourteen, I was at an appointment with Marley when the doctor started to talk about next steps and the need for dialysis to be considered. I had no idea what was going on. It sounded horrifying that I would have to rely on a machine to keep me alive, and how far I would have to travel for treatment. I checked out mentally and stared down at my jumper, which I remember had tassels that I started playing with to avoid this hideous and heavy conversation. There were four of us in the consulting room – me, Marley, a nurse and the doctor. I was white-faced, silent and obstinately tight lipped, not able to comprehend what this could mean for me. Marley and the nurse were in tears. I felt like I needed to hold my own and just take in the news. I thought, I'll take it like a hard brick wall and show no emotion because I'm FINE. I felt annoyed at the tears of the others. I didn't cry, although all I wanted to do was howl. Howl from my very belly. What was I to do? What did this mean for me? All these questions that I had no idea how to begin to even form, let alone give a voice to.

There are two types of dialysis treatments: one is the haemodialysis (HD) (haemo means blood, so it is also known as blood dialysis) and the other is peritoneal dialysis (PD), which is done via an abdominal catheter. The peritoneum membrane is used as a filter for toxins, through a glucose solution placed inside the abdomen and then drained out. HD uses an artificial kidney: through needling, blood comes out, through the artificial kidney and back into the body, and takes four to six hours per session. PD uses osmosis and diffusion.

It is a longer treatment, at eight hours a night. The nurse spoke to Marley separately after this appointment and counselled her that the HD option would be better for me, as having an abdominal catheter at age fourteen could cause body embarrassment issues.

I was not party to that initial decision and am glad, in hindsight, that it was made for me as I think, based on me being so young, it was the better option. And inherently, without question, I trusted my mother to make the best, intuitive decision for me

We left the appointment to come home, and I felt a combination of terrible sadness and considerable rage. I banged the door shut to the bathroom where I sat and cried and cried. I don't remember much about the rest of the unfolding after that. My parents and I went to a private meeting with my then GP, a lovely, bearded family man, who offered this meeting at his home, to discuss the next steps. They wanted to admit me to hospital again for heavy doses of steroids, which I did not want. I wished to stay at home, so I took the steroids without going to hospital. This course of heavy duty steroids did nothing to help and, some weeks after, I was hospitalised in Portsmouth, a long way from our home in Dorchester.

Whilst in hospital, I remember my parents coming to visit. And how very tired Parley looked. The doctors gave them, rather than me, my diagnosis of chronic renal failure. It was as if I was just an appendage, lying in the hospital bed. Around that time, I was fitted with a sub-clavian catheter (a tube to the side of the collarbone), in order to be dialysed. I had a fistula created in my left arm, which takes a few weeks to mature to be safely needled. Not much of this was really fully explained to me, so I felt I was being man-handled most of the time, just a body moving through these dark and difficult experiences. I was so glad to come home.

When I came home from hospital after this episode, I recall sitting on the toilet and the sub-clavian catheter literally sliding out of me. It seemed my body was done with it, so I did not need the additional procedure usually required to remove it. The catheter had been inserted for quicker access to dialyse, which had been needed on admission to hospital. I still remember the doctor who fitted it, as she kept calling me poppet during the procedure, and silent tears rolled down my face. I also had surgery to join a vein and artery together in my left arm, creating the fistula. It buzzed, as there was blood moving through it at such force. This is the intention, as it creates a strong vessel that can then be needled to act as an important access site for haemodialysis.

All this treatment took place on an adult ward 75 miles away from home, where I had to face all these experiences alone. It was only a much more recent conversation with Marley that revealed how she had felt coming to visit me one day and discovering I'd had the fistula operation. She said she was horrified, as she'd had no idea it had happened and never got over that news, because of all that it represented.

Once my treatment started, there was so much to adapt to. I had fluid and dietary restrictions, as well as having to spend two nights away from home each week in the Portsmouth dialysis unit. Again, this was on an adult ward, which I'm not sure is the best place for a fourteen year old girl. I was the youngest there and had no peer-to-peer support. It felt like I was the only young person going through this bleak journey. Some nights on the dialysis machine I would have to sleep in a chair, as beds were not always available. I would go deeply inwards for these sessions and didn't exert my personality. It felt easier to just shut down mentally, let the treatment be done, and walk away from the unit and leave it behind me until next time. I could then ease back into my usual bright and lively self, bring that side of me to school, relax with my parents and just be me. At this time my regime was six-hour treatments, twice weekly. Some sessions on the machine would be non-eventful, but some were very upsetting if the nurse wasn't good at needling – there could be a 'blow out' where the vessel is missed, leading to a significant internal tissue bleed. Some days my whole arm would be black and blue, from the top of my shoulder, all the way down to the wrist. Thankfully, this was rare. In other sessions, too much fluid was taken off; in my dehydrated state, my blood pressure would drop severely and I would almost black out. As time went by, I adapted and started to get to know my physical responses, in terms of what was the right amount of fluid to programme the machine to remove. Whilst I mentally shut down to the external world, I was razor clear internally and observed everything. That skill has stayed with me. It's very useful when I am very ill and at the perceived mercy of nurses and doctors. I can still be aware of what feels right for me.

Of course, there's nothing natural about dialysis and it's not normal to have your blood outside of your body, so there were a number of different side effects. One still has high levels of nitrogenous waste cycling through the blood, but at levels that are just about manageable. One remains in renal failure and all the complications that come with that. This means it's not a great long-term treatment. This form of dialysis treatment effectively puts the kidneys into shock, and in most cases patients usually cease producing urine, as happened to me a few weeks after commencing treatment. This required a strict fluid restriction, an enormous challenge as I was limited to just half a litre of fluid a day, which was extremely difficult. Imagine just having a bowl of soup and a glass of water! That would be your fluid restriction filled for the whole day. It's important to adhere to it as much as possible because, if you don't, fluid accumulates in the body which the machine then has to be programmed to remove. Over time this builds up, and extraction puts great strain on the heart. I witnessed people who would come in severely overloaded with fluid and were regularly having three to four litres of fluid removed. I felt it was important to manage this. But it was very hard, and I didn't always. Sometimes I would obsess in my mind about having a cool, long glass of water or be able to drink endless mugs of tea.

I came to know which nurses I liked and were skilled at needling. There was a push rather quickly for me to get involved in setting up the trolley and laying out the needles and other ancillary equipment needed for my treatment. I would see other patients resist this and want to have everything done for them, but I realised contributing in this way was helpful to me and the nurses.

I felt much more content living back with my own family. Marley did her best to take me to practitioners who might be able to help me with my health. I went for allergy testing, homeopathy and saw a healer. The latter actually came in and visited me at home after I had started haemodialysis.

Whilst there was no sudden healing episode of my kidneys regaining function, these healing sessions did offer me an opportunity to self-soothe and to trust - and, indeed, feel - supported. I have come to realise now, of course, that healing happens in many forms.

What is important to emphasise here is that dialysis is no like-for-like match for our own clever and amazing kidneys. The treatments can extract some waste and excess fluid, but in truth it performs only about ten per cent of what our own kidneys do. So what do your kidneys do for you? Some of the functions may surprise you. They are important regulators of our haemoglobin as they produce the hormone erythropoetin, so help prevent anaemia. As a result, anaemia and fatigue can be commonplace with impaired kidney function. They also help regulate blood pressure, making it key to manage a healthy blood pressure to protect the kidneys. If the pressure is too high, it can damage the millions of tiny glomeruli, the kidney's tiny filters. They also co-ordinate with the para-thyroid glands located in the throat, to aid healthy bone mineralisation. In addition, they produce bicarbonate, so act as a valuable buffering system in maintaining the internal acid/alkali balance. Therefore, metabolic acidosis can be associated with impaired kidney function which is not, by any means, a thriving cellular situation. So you can appreciate, when the kidneys go offline, the knock-on medical impact is considerable. And that's without talking about the deeper spiritual and emotional qualities of the kidneys. As much as technology has advanced, it can't replicate the splendour and infinite wisdom of nature in the structure of our own anatomy.

In the initial years on haemodialysis, I was very resistant to having a transplant. I felt I wanted to keep giving my kidneys the chance to wake up. The thought of a transplant was really quite alien, even frightening. I had an instinct of how difficult such an invasive surgery would be: I'd lose my figure, the drug regime would be punishing, and I felt it would be a long and painful recovery.

But then when I was about seventeen, I had a change of heart. I happened upon a television programme covering the Transplant Games and thought, 'Wow! You can still be active and do stuff after having a transplant!'. So, I agreed to go on the transplant list. About three years had gone by before I made this decision. It was a big breakthrough and Marley was thrilled at the news. My family had respected my previous decision not to have a transplant, and it was very much a no-go area of discussion. In fact any suggestion of this would make me very angry, as I'd felt strongly I wanted to heal my own kidneys. A fellow patient, who travelled in the volunteer car with me from Dorchester to Portsmouth for a while, got the call for a kidney and I went to visit her after her surgery. I remember telling her I was going to heal my own kidneys, so didn't need a transplant. When I told Marley that this lady was no longer travelling with me as she had a new kidney, she gently said, "Wouldn't you consider it?" at which I flew into a rage, and stormed off.

At the same time I went on the transplant list, I decided to become more involved with my own medical care. A fellow male patient played a big role in this decision, as he chatted to me about how he did his own needling. He was a big, gentle giant of a man with smiley eyes, and I admired how at ease he was with everything. So, I learned how to needle myself: two big needles into the fistula, one to take blood out and circulate it into the artificial kidney and the other to return the filtered blood back in. I was good at it! I did not even need the lignocane anaesthetic prior to the needle insertion, which was standard, and actually creates a lot of the scar tissue. The seed for this had been planted on a girls' holiday to Spain when I was at university, where the medics did not use the anaesthetic and my Spanish nurse said it added to the scar tissue more than the needles themselves. This kind of information matters and it had taken four years for me to hear it. For the remaining three years I was on this form of treatment and doing my own needle insertion, minimal scar tissue built up on my left arm. Once involved in my own treatment, I learned how to set up the machine and take myself on and off. I took my own blood pressure, wrote down my observations, and felt much more in control. This was incredibly empowering. At one point, when things were just a bit hectic, I was even asked to take another patient's blood pressure! It was a good feeling to be relied upon and trusted, even at just seventeen years old.

Outside of my treatment, I got excellent GCSE grades, was the Deputy Head Girl at my school, and achieved the right A levels to get me into my university of choice, Royal Holloway, part of the University of London.

I skipped off to study with some moments of trepidation, as it would mean making a new set of friends and explaining why I disappeared three times a week. At this stage, I was extremely private about my health issues. My close group of friends from school were incredibly supportive, but it had taken some time for me to open up about my situation. Once they knew, it was no big deal. But even then, I still never really talked about it, or how I was feeling. As I went for dialysis on a Friday night, we had our night out on a Saturday, and there was no sense of me missing out.

I had a blast at university, and my initial jitters soon dissipated as I experienced a new set of lovely friends. I got the precious gift of a car from my parents in my second year, so could drive myself to and from dialysis treatments. This gave me a sense of freedom and a relief from relying on hospital transport, which I had used in my first year of study. I remember feeling utterly mortified being picked up in a car with a 'Hospital Transport' sign in the front window. What if a boy I fancied saw me!

Although still young, I had a clear sense of celebrating the small victories and moments. For example, a satellite dialysis unit was opened up in Woking so during my final year at university, my commute for treatments was only about twenty minutes, versus the previous forty-five it had been to Carshalton. It was also a smaller set up and the three nurses who ran it were utterly adorable. We could order a sandwich of our choice and it would be freshly made for us and brought on a proper china plate, with a cup of tea served in cup and saucer. These simple little things brought me great comfort and I felt much more myself in this setting. I remember one day being really stressed about being so tired, with exams looming and feeling overwhelmed. Unusually, I had a cry during the dialysis session while talking to the lovely nurse, Emma, who was so sweet and just said, "Do you have a friend you can talk to?" So, afterwards, I drove to see my friend Ed. Reminders to reach out are useful.

By this time, the dialysis treatments had increased to three times weekly for better health. It was when I was doing my A-levels and dialysing in Oxford that the nurses suggested increasing my twice weekly treatments. I was concerned: mostly, I didn't want to be more of a burden to my family, who were driving me back and forth for treatment, as I wasn't keen to rely on hospital transport again. But we made it work, and between my parents and my sister, who had since graduated and was working in Oxford, I was very grateful to have that taxi support! I did feel a lot healthier with the three weekly sessions, as there was less of a gap between blood filtering and less toxins had built up. Together with me being able to drive myself there and back, this was an overall improvement. In addition, as my treatment was more regular, the hours on the machine were reduced to three to four hour sessions, which felt much more manageable segments of time compared to six hours.

I certainly embraced my wild side at university. I did drink alcohol, probably too much for my situation, and had everyone drinking vodka and lime - as I found it was not too much fluid, and would get you pretty drunk! I did not have clear awareness of my limits and as well as drinking, I was quite promiscuous. It was a fantastical side I developed, as it presented freedom. I wanted to be a carefree young woman who could do what she wanted and be desirable. Of course, this was not the truth, as I would never tell these boys about myself and I would hope they wouldn't notice the buzzing in my arm from the fistula. I was just a wild girl. Anyone that showed a true interest, I would push away. I almost felt it was ridiculous someone could love me for who I really was, and I also felt I really needed to manage the health situation on my own. Whilst I might have believed this was me being independent it was, of course, a fear of intimacy. Getting close to someone would mean opening up about what I had to endure and how I felt about it all. My darling friend Ed fell in love with me and I just could not return the feelings. I said no to any possibilities for true intimacy and continued to draw in good looking, one-night stands that were, in truth, meaningless - but made me feel better about myself.

In my final year at university, I got a call from a doctor at my Oxford hospital. He said, "Ummm, I can't find your name on the transplant list." Two years had gone since I'd made the decision to have a transplant. "Oh," I said. It seemed the angst to proceed to be listed had culminated in a mistake. Or so it seemed. I was amused rather than upset by this, as I already had an understanding that dramatising situations helps little. By now I was nineteen, five years on dialysis. I didn't feel angry at this mistake. I didn't even ask how it had happened. I just trusted it would be corrected.

One other option is live donor kidney donation, which is a very valuable and precious source of organ transplantation. But how does anyone ask another human for a kidney? It has to be offered from a place of true love and care. I was very clear in my own mind that I simply could not accept a kidney from someone living. It was not meant to be my path. When we were younger, my sister sent me a letter when she was away at university, offering me one of her kidneys. However, funnily enough we always thought we had different blood types so I told her she was off the hook! It was not until many years later it transpired we were the same blood group. Parley is the same blood group as me, but he was very clear he did not want to donate as he wanted me to have the best opportunity to have a good quality kidney. He felt he was too old and I entirely respected that.

In truth, I was relieved I did not need to ask this of my dear family, who already had dealt with a lot on this journey.

At a party one Saturday night during sixth form, where a little booze had been drunk and people were a bit tipsy, the conversation turned to my situation. This prompted one friend to say, "Can we all get tested to see if we're a match?" I had a lovely group of girlfriends from sixth form and it was a very touching moment. One friend deliberately pulled me aside and offered me a kidney. I felt unable to accept or even seriously entertain any of this. I remained clear in my mind that it wasn't the option for me, as it just felt like too much to ask of someone. Even when it is offered from a place of love and care, there has to be a willingness to accept from the person in need. So when that happens, it's a wonderful thing. Doctors and transplant coordinators play a role in steering this conversation, too. My friend Anoushica, whose brother gave her a kidney, was also horrified at the initial thought of needing a kidney transplant following a lupus diagnosis and very serious illness. The consultant on the ward talked to her family and set the scene for a solution of a live donor kidney. As a result of that sensitive conversation, Anoushica's boyfriend, brother and another friend came forward to be tested. A supported conversation helped. It facilitated practicality.

Amazingly, there are also altruistic donors who give a kidney to a stranger. The topic is now a lot more openly talked about than before, and I have seen the conversation evolve more widely over the years.

Because I am exposed to so much through my regular visits to hospital and am now involved as a peer supporter, I have opened my heart much more to all the wonderful and moving stories I hear, about what people do for their loved ones.

And so from young childhood, through difficult teen years into young adulthood, these were my formative years.

That little, healthy girl, growing up under the Zambian sky, knew how magical and beautiful the earth really was. She carried me through my very difficult teenage experiences, and was open to the healing capacity of friendship, family and laughter. She trusted Professor Thompson, because there was no other way he made her feel but trusted and safe. She knew in her soul the capacity humanity has to heal, in spite of the storms.

She became the woman I am today and my I love her for it.

My fervent hope is that my experiences help you to awaken your inner physician, in ways that serve your unique journey towards being wholly aligned within yourself and within your life path. I have so many tools to share with you. Along with the power of story and practical advice, I wish to add value to your health and wellbeing.

Let it be so.

Aho we exclaim together, with our arms outstretched to the skies and our faces turned towards the sun.

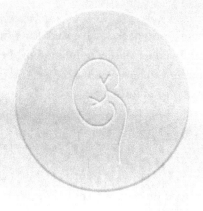

CHAPTER TWO

Along comes Kenny Kidney

A single phone call on 14th October 1997 changed the course of my life.

It was from the transplant co-ordinator, telling me they had a kidney for me. The hospital had been trying to reach me for hours (no prevalent ownership of mobile phones at that time) and were about to call the police to enlist their help. I was living at home with my parents following my graduation that summer, and was working in an office with Marley. She had left earlier to go home and called me to say there was a voicemail to call the hospital. This meant I was on my own when I got the news. I wandered into the office next door in a kind of daze saying, "They have a kidney for me."

"Sit down, sit down," they cried. I sat. But Cripes! I had to go. I had no time to sit!

I returned home from work, packed a bag and drove myself the half hour drive to the hospital. I said to Marley to tell no-one, in case it was a false alarm and turned out not to be a match after all. This does happen and I'd seen some fellow patients go through this over the years. I felt incredibly calm driving there. I had to check myself into the hospital. "What are you here for?" the administrator asked. "I'm here for a new kidney." It was surreal.

I reflect sometimes upon the man who gifted me his kidney, through the agreement of his family. I think of him as a little boy, growing up and living his life and what a beautiful, beautiful gift his passing gave to me. I can get very emotional about it, because it is so beautiful. I think of both of us as innocent children and how little we knew how our paths would converge many years into the future, on such an intimate level. Through kidney transplantation, I get to experience a relationship beyond time-bound human interaction. I've never met this man, yet part of his physical form is now inside of me and part of me. It is a gift out of linear time, it came in a wave from the realm of Spirit. It took many years for the connection to be made and was exactly the one I was meant to receive. To me, it is a true representation of how deeply connected we all are.

Arriving at the transplant ward, I introduced myself. It felt strange having never before taken the turn to enter this ward, but it was finally my time to go that way. The transplant coordinator, Kevin, called me princess and had a very kind manner about him. I was meeting a lot of new people for the first time, in a life-changing circumstance. All the while, I still felt incredibly calm, taking it all in. I asked Kevin if it was a good match, and he smiled and said yes. I had bloods drawn to confirm this was still the case, along with a number of pre-surgery diagnostic tests. A young male, red-headed doctor, wearing black rimmed, glasses, greeted me to do the ECG. It was cold enough being mid-October, but I had to undress my top half, breasts bare, to fit the electrodes. The doctor made me feel very at ease and chatted away without it feeling awkward. I had a dialysis session on the usual day ward I attended to ensure blood was as clean as it could be pre-op. Although I had said to Marley that I didn't want a fuss, once I knew it was going ahead, I called as many friends, whose telephone numbers I knew by heart, as I could. There were tears, there were high emotions, all of them saying, "I'm coming to see you as soon as possible." We love you. I know. Oh my, I know. I felt supported and safe. There was no trepidation.

I had called home to confirm to my parents that it was a green light. I said: "Remember, no fuss please. See you on the other side." But, of course, they're my people, my blood, my family and my support, so they came to the dialysis ward later that evening, my folks and my sister. It was a heartwarming moment seeing them all walk in together with big smiles on their faces, as if they were saying, "Seriously, did you think we wouldn't come?"

The surgeon came to check me out. This was the first time I'd met him. He came across as even tempered, very direct and efficient in a polite way – a quiet, diligent and safe man. When I had finished the dialysis session, I was given the first dose of immuno-suppressant drugs back on the transplant ward. I remember I was worried the high dose of steroids would have an effect immediately and asked the nurse if my face was starting to swell! She reassured me it would take a few days for them to kick in. In a moment I remember so clearly, I took a bath and remember standing up, completely naked after bathing and looking at my full reflection in the mirror saying to myself, "This is where it all changes, Ciara. This is it." Naked, closing this current chapter, about to slide into the next one.

It was into the early hours of the following morning when I was taken up for surgery. I was sleepy and had started to fall asleep whilst waiting. In cases of cadaveric donor organs, time of death cannot be anticipated so the surgical team does need to be able to operate as swiftly as possible in order to give the organ the best chance to thrive. Blessed be these surgical teams who work around the clock.

My sister had called late into the night. I stood in the middle of the ward at the phone on reception, taking the call. She was crying, "Remember, I love you."

"I know," I said. "I love you too."

And so, with that love and support in my belly, stripped bare and in my attractive hospital attire, I was ready. After about four hours of surgery, I groggily came around in recovery. I had a new kidney grafted into my left iliac crest.

"How's Kenny?" Aisling asked as she came into my room when she visited me the next day.

"Who is Kenny?" I enquired through my drugged and dazed state, hooked up to an oxygen machine, a urinary catheter and on pain control medicine.

Kenny kidney. Ah. And Kenny was named. And what a marvellous Kenny he was.

I was in hospital for about ten days. My close friends came zooming in with armloads of gifts, including a huge teddy bear I named Kev, after the transplant coordinator. Magazines, puzzle books, get well balloons. So many visitors. So much love. So many good wishes. Cards from relatives, with thoughtful messages. The staff were all lovely. I really warmed to my surgeon. An apparently reserved man with a very kind and a simple manner, and a sense of humour. No ego. He recommended cranberry juice, which made me like him even more for sharing such a useful piece of advice.

The young, red-headed doctor came by a couple of evenings and played backgammon with me on his later shifts, which I felt comforted by. It was rare to have such simple kindness and companionship in a hospital from a doctor. It was sweet.

I had some fun experiences on the ward over those ten days. Aisling came in every evening with food (hospital food is no good). She was still living in Oxford, a very short distance from the hospital. One evening she arrived with a cracking headache. I told her to lie down on my bed and I sat in the bedside chair, and asked the nurse for some painkillers to help my sister. She reluctantly agreed, as medications were not meant for anyone other than the patient. I also remember the nurses from the Woking dialysis unit sent me flowers. It was only fairly recently, after I had graduated, that I stopped going there for dialysis, so I had called them a few days post-surgery to tell them the happy news. Unfortunately, they had to be given away as fresh flowers are an infection risk and cannot be kept on transplant wards.

Another day, when I was able to move around a little better, the ward was under-staffed and the matron asked me to 'cover the phones'. So I sat in my pyjamas and answered the phone, helping and taking messages where I could. We laughed about it, imagining the tabloid headline: 'Patient Made to Work Whilst Recovering from Major Surgery!' I was happy to do it. It was human helping human. And it made me feel useful.

I didn't poo the first few days after surgery – as you can imagine, a combination of general anaesthetic, recovery and an extra organ being inside me made a smooth bowel movement tricky! And I didn't want to force it and burst open my stitches! However, the threat of suppositories soon got things moving.

Being twenty-one, I had the benefit of youth on my side. As is often the case, Kenny kidney took a little while to settle in, so initially I was still having dialysis sessions. My friend Vivien, who had her transplant a couple of years ahead of me, reassured me that although kidneys can work immediately in the surgery, it was normal for a kidney to take a little while to get going. Finally, after about a week, and seven years on haemodialysis, my kidney function was at a level that required no more dialysis. My goodness. The kidney was working very well. Our human ability to adapt to our circumstances is so strong. Whilst this was all very exciting and everyone was thrilled, there was still a fairly long period of recovery and adaptation. The flip side was a huge drug regime, especially at the beginning when I was taking about ten different drugs. Three of those were specific to immuno-suppression.

I was urinating quite regularly as my bladder adapted to carrying urine again. At first, I would get the urge to wee every hour as it got used to being used for the first time in seven years!

A great piece of fortune and synchronicity was that my sister was living about a ten-minute walk from the hospital in Oxford. Again, life brings us what we need. I appreciated being able to stay with her and her housemates, as I could just get on with my recovery in the peace of a lovely house, when Aisling and her housemates were out at work. I liked being able to potter about without anyone fussing, but there was a youthful, exuberant energy around me when everyone arrived home for the evenings. It was a period that cemented a great closeness between my sister and me. She really was my rock during that time. We even found humour in some of the downsides of the transplant. I started calling myself the bearded lady, as I experienced increased hair growth as a result of the drugs I was taking. Thankfully, the hospital provided electrolysis for female patients. The growth wasn't horrendous, but it was noticeable enough to make me self-conscious. However, I also realised it was a small price to pay for the upside of having kidney function again.

A close eye is kept at the beginning to watch for any sign of organ rejection or infection, but luckily I could easily walk to and from the hospital without needing to rely on anyone else. That felt like freedom.

Especially after having to rely on my parents and my sister as volunteer drivers for so long. And I'd had to rely on the dialysis machine. Although I had waited many years for this, I knew this kidney was the one for me. It felt safe in my body. I laughed so much. I would spend long periods of time just laughing. I'd always been someone who embraced silliness and giggles, but this really ramped up during my healing time. However, I had to modify my laugh so it was wide, open-mouthed and silent, as a proper belly laughing was too much for the scar and my healing tissues!

I had a great appetite. A combination of feeling overall better, but another side effect of the steroids, which I was taking for immune-suppression purposes. I merrily ate three meals a day.

After two months of recovery, I felt it was time to return to work and moved back home to my parents. In hindsight, this was perhaps a bit premature. Not long after, when I was still adjusting to the side effects of the medication, I stopped passing urine. Clearly this was extremely worrying. I went into the hospital where a catheter was fitted directly into the kidney, so urine could drain out. It transpired the kidney's ureter –the tube connected to the kidney so urine can drain into the bladder – had died off.

Over the next few weeks, I had various scans to assess what was going on. During one of them I caught an infection, which must have come from the catheter being uncovered for too long, and felt completely awful. Raging temperature and headache. Shivers. So back to the ward it was, as I couldn't keep anything down – including the drugs – so these had to be administered intravenously. Having a bad infection when you are already recovering from intense surgery, and being immuno-suppressed, is not ideal. I was discharged after a couple of days and once again returned to recover at my sister's place. All of this was draining and disappointing. It also seemed to be taking so long for a solution to be decided. First there was talk of putting in a stent, but then further surgery was decided.

So, close to Christmas, just over two months after the transplant, I was re-admitted for a second surgery to move one of my native ureters and connect it to the kidney. The right solution, but it meant another four or five hours of surgery. Another recovery.

As it was coming up to Christmas, the nurses got gifts for the patients. I got a Tigger – one of those beanie characters, only little – but so cute. I sat him on my bedside table and on one of the surgeon's rounds he started to play with him. A young nurse looked at me and we exchanged a glance of humour as we asked the surgeon if he was ok! It was another sweet moment. The surgeon seemed quite taken with Tigger.

The second surgery was successful and performed by the same lovely surgeon who had done the transplant, and he also tied off my fistula when I asked for that to be done. No more buzzing in my arm.

As the surgeon had been so taken by Tigger, I went to the Disney store and got one for him as a thank you. I gave it to the same nurse who had been with me when he started playing with it at my bedside, to pass onto him. She thought it was a lovely gesture, telling me that surgeons rarely get gifts, which mostly go to the nurses. A few weeks later I received a very formal looking letter from the hospital . It was a thank you letter from the surgeon, saying Tigger had successfully joined the transplant surgery team and was getting along very well, in spite of his small stature! That made me smile from my very heart.

I went on to have another fifteen years of great kidney function, was in largely good health, and had no hospital stays. I learned how to listen deeply to my body. From the very beginning, I instinctively felt I was on too much immuno-suppression. I came across a letter many years later which I'd written to the head professor at The Churchill in Oxford, asking when could I come off the steroids and reduce the cyclosporin dose. I smiled at the tenacity of my younger self. I went travelling around the world a year after having the transplant. When I came back, I was able to tail off the steroids to nil, which was the protocol at the Oxford hospital. Over the course of the next few years I also stopped one of the other drugs, called azathioprine. I was going on holiday to Australia and knew I'd be getting a lot of sun exposure so wanted to reduce risk of skin damage, and I viewed being on less immune suppression as more protective to my skin. When I returned back to London, it did not feel necessary to resume taking it. My bloods continued to be excellent and I had also come across articles written in the USA on the benefits of mono-therapy – single drug therapy for immuno-suppression. This is essentially where I had gravitated to, following my own intuition.

I shared with the renal team that I was only taking cyclosporin after about a year, as I felt confident there was a track record and evidence that this mono-therapy approach was working for me. And the team accepted this without issue, although I was reminded not to cease the drugs altogether.

The approach of suppressing the immune system so a donor organ is not rejected has its validity, yet it is also very reductionist. The immune system is highly complex and individual for each person. We all respond differently to our environment, to our emotions, to our food. The danger in organ donation lies in the inflammatory cascade being triggered. And interestingly, this complex inflammatory cascade is the driver of most diseases.

At this stage I had just donated a considerable amount of blood, as I was participating in a research study on what is termed 'tolerance'. The reason I had been asked was because I was now fully drug free, a very unusual anomaly within the transplant patient community. This followed a very gradual, full tailing off of the one final drug I had remained on, cyclosporin, knowing my blood work continued to be excellent. I had heard nothing about this research before being asked to donate blood and later discovered it had been ongoing for about ten years. This both thrilled and fascinated me: the idea that I was able to contribute, in a meaningful way, to a better drug regime for patients and potentially - for some - even no drugs at all, if their markers for tolerance could be properly interpreted. This was extremely exciting. I felt like there was a bigger picture as to why I had been intuitively drawn to coming off all medication.

Through this I was invited to an evening where the multi-disciplinary team were presenting their research and the detail of their findings. I feel this door would never have been open to me if I had not taken the route of drug cessation. It expanded my experience and I was exposed to information I never would have been otherwise. Most significant were the stories the team told. One of the nephrologists spoke about the time they realised some patients could cease their medication. The story began in Poland, where a man's home was flooded and he ended up getting stuck upstairs. He was a transplant recipient taking the required immuno-suppression. However, the medication was in his now flooded downstairs. Some days passed and by the time he was rescued, although very stressed, tests showed there was no indication of any damage to the transplant kidney. This story prompted research into why some patients could cease medications and others could not. During this evening I heard many more stories like this, which I was intrigued by. There were a number of other transplant patients in attendance, some with their partners or family members. I came alone, as I like to do in these situations so I can focus. One gentleman spoke about how he had been diagnosed with cancer and the prognosis was not good. After discussion with his doctor, it was suggested he stop the immuno-suppression and watch and see what might happen, given there was nothing to lose. It was high risk, but also worth it if things stayed stable with both the kidney and the cancer reverses. Which is what happened. Amazing, right? These are tense and very personal situations and, as such, it has to be for the patient to decide what to do. This man was now several years cancer free as his own immune system was able to handle it and he seemed to have the markers for tolerance that made it safe for him to cease the drugs.

In Christmas 2012, I had an inflammatory event in my right big toe joint. This hadn't happened before and as a nutritionist and yoga teacher, I was perplexed as to why it had occurred. It was extremely painful and I could not put weight on it for some days. At the time I thought it was due to the excesses of the festive season, and did not realise that something more pervasive and systemic was in progress.

At my regular follow up in transplant clinic the next month, my blood pressure had risen considerably to 150/100. I was also leaking protein in my urine and my blood creatinine level – one measure of kidney function – had crept up. Collectively, all these signs did not bode well for the kidney. He was starting to struggle and I was feeling it.

This inflammatory toe event marked the beginning of a substantial decline in kidney function. I was advised by the renal team to resume triple immuno-suppression, which I did. I had always taken a very practical view and was willing to accept this drug resumption. However, I did not really feel the approach was particularly creative, especially as my regular doctor did not think it was rejection. I had two kidney biopsies over the course of a few weeks to help understand what might be going on. However, what I wasn't told was that the biopsy results would not be conclusive, and there was a disagreement within my medical team about whether it was rejection or a recurrence of the glomerular nephritis - the original cause of the renal failure in my own kidneys, years previously - or, indeed, something else. This was further complicated by two doctors saying it was not behaving like a typical episode of rejection, which was backed up by my main doctor who just did not feel it was. I could feel the discord rising within the medical community about my case. I felt for my doctor, as she was the interface to what I imagine was a strong wall of resistance from the other consultants. I did not feel well. My body was struggling with the considerable decline in kidney function, along with all the stress of being in and out of the renal unit. I had not anticipated this outcome, and I had to face a lot fears and a lot of old patterns. What was I ready to deal with?

How would it feel to have to resume dialysis? I had to really explore dark places and crevices and old stuff I had never really processed when I was young. I had to go deep - and there was no option to turn away from how I was feeling.

I continued to feel for my doctor. I could sense she was under enormous pressure, and she was calling me regularly to talk about my results and potential next steps. I also now recognise that she also probably felt partly responsible, as she'd previously asked me to take part in tolerance studies and sharing stories of other patients who had ceased their drug regimes, albeit for very specific reasons.

At the second biopsy, as the renal function was so low, the protocol was to administer a synthetic form of anti-diuretic hormone called vasopressin. The possible side effects of this were not explained to me and two days after this biopsy, I felt dreadful. I had not experienced this after the first biopsy, so had no reason to look out for certain symptoms. I really thought it was curtains for the kidney. I was puffy and my blood pressure was elevated. The consensus amongst the consultants was this was rejection and that pulsed intravenous steroids were necessary. Feeling horrid, I went into hospital the next day for what I had thought was simply going to be a conversation, only to be rushed in and a doctor I did not know very well was saying, "We need to get this under control," in a panicked way. Bloods were taken and then, without any conversation, I was hooked up for the first dose of IV steroids. I felt it necessary because I was so unwell.

What had actually happened is the synthetic antidiuretic hormone had caused hyponatremia, meaning my sodium levels had fallen to a dangerous level. As a key electrolyte, when this happens it can lead to a coma. I only know this is what happened after looking up my own results online at a later date. No doctor picked this up in the panic to give me the steroids at the time, and the protocol of administering massive pulsed steroids to a patient in hyponatremia is questionable. My regular doctor told me later this had happened to another lady who then passed out at home on her own, luckily to be found by her son. I personally question the use of this drug as standard protocol. It is administered prior to a kidney biopsy, when the GFR (glomerular filtration rate) of the patient is below a certain percentage, arguably putting more pressure on the kidney and endocrine system. When I asked why this drug is still used, the response was quite vague. As sometimes happens in medicine, something gets used once as an idea and then becomes standard protocol.

Probably one of the lowest points in all of this was finding out that the kidney function had worsened after three massive doses of steroids. They had not helped and further threw off my blood pressure. This was a big blow. I remember sitting alone, processing this on my sofa, feeling a dense knot in the very pit of my stomach. My usual doctor called with the results, and she started to go through all the other results aside from the creatinine. I knew she was building up for bad news. The kidney function had further deteriorated, leaving very little room for much more decline. Dread. Disappointment. Despair. Dear God, let this not swallow me up. Give me strength to lift out of this. Is this the end?

To clarify with regards the immune suppression drugs, I was sporadically taking cyclosporin for about seven years and then entirely drug free for about two, which was a meaningful length of time. My labs continued to be good and actually showed slight improvement. This made sense, as ironically, the immuno-suppressive drugs are in fact nephrotoxic – meaning that, over time, they cause damage to the renal tissue. This is an issue for all transplant patients: if you have had a heart or liver transplant, for example, the drugs can damage the native kidneys too. A father of my friend was one of the first heart transplant recipients and had a fabulous few decades with the donor heart. However, he experienced kidney failure due to the drugs. I am quite sure many precautions can be taken to minimise this damage, but people need access to the information. They need to know about good hydration with good quality water, a whole food diet, to avoid processed food and take excellent liver tonics, such as plentiful garlic and turmeric. They also need a spiritual practice to help face the ongoing challenges that arise with transplantation.

Whilst it is a tremendous gift, to receive a donor organ it is not a journey without challenge.

Kenny kidney offered me so many years of health, where I travelled widely, built a successful career, fell in love and was engaged to be married, and bought my own home. On the surface, what a great life! And yes, it was - in many, many ways. But how much had I truly awakened my inner physician to her full potential?

During the time when the kidney function held at circa eighteen per cent, there was not really much room for further decline. However, amazingly, it stabilised there. This stability became my utmost focus. For me, eighteen per cent was enough. Enough to still have freedom. My doctor said some people stay at this level for years, so I felt heartened that I could adapt, I could use this time as an opportunity to help myself on all levels. To self-care. To discover more ways to feel my way back to wellness.

I reached out to find ways to help myself. I started working with an energy healer, who helped me enormously and would push me at times to consider how I really felt. This all became the greatest gift. It was a reassessment, a realignment. I found a naturopathic doctor in the USA, who had also been through kidney failure and transplantation and was, at that time, back on haemodialysis. This helped me to see more clearly that no matter what, there are always ways to take responsibility and to self-care. I started having regular bodywork with a super Thai massage therapist. I went off and did a 10-day Vipassana, a completely silent meditation retreat, where we did about ten hours of meditation daily with no distractions, not even reading a book. I also stopped drinking alcohol during this period. I began to connect with my own meditation practice at home. I completed a number of 40-day mantra cycles to keep centred and connected.

This was a massive awakening for me. I thought I had been awake, but there was more to go. It was another initiation into releasing fears and setting new, healthier patterns. I was so grateful for it. How else, I wonder, could I have found my way? How else could I truly understand what it is to be fully alive? It was my journey. My unfolding. I was still well enough to travel and over the following three years, I made the most of it. I spent time with my cousin Lisa in Los Angeles, I visited my precious friend Dana in Oaxaca, Mexico. I completed my 500-hour yoga training in the Andes, near Cusco in Peru. And then back to the States to herald in the new year of 2016, in beautiful Sedona with Lisa.

The brick walls I had spent years constructing and maintaining were still there, but as my kidney function declined they began to lose their strength. I started to talk a lot more with my closest friends and my dear Marley about how I was feeling, and saying out loud the word dialysis – something I had never wanted to consider again.

I remember after one doctor's appointment, standing in the middle of Crystal Palace on the phone to Marley, crying. Well, sobbing, actually, but also starting to accept that it would be ok, whatever happened. Marley shared with me on that call how she had listened to a radio interview with a lady who'd had four kidney transplants. This was a turning point for me towards acceptance and, indeed, gratitude that I had options. I could pursue another kidney and that was ok. But I had to explore that intimacy with reality. I thought, here I am, this is now, I can navigate these experiences.

I started to properly review my relationship dynamics with men as well. It took me about five years to recover from a heart-breaking end to my most significant long-term relationship many years earlier, where both of us had abandonment issues. During those years, I self-sabotaged a lot. I attracted superficial characters, or people who talked about themselves, which allowed me to not have to reveal myself emotionally. On the surface I was very confident, but I kept repeating these patterns and would be broken after each situation. Men needing rescuing kept coming my way, because I had not taken the time to honestly consider: what did I want? None of them knew anything about my health situation as I did not talk about it. This awakening needed to impact my whole life, not just my health.

The danger comes when the more you wish to reassure others and not be a burden, the more you neglect your own needs. This whole protracted kidney transplant rejection episode, no matter how stark and difficult it was, asked me to turn towards my deep-seated fears and look at them. From a place of compassion for my own experience, I was able to do this. All of this allowed me the space to reflect and explore previous relationship patterns. I came to realise that the pattern of fixing and healing my partner provided me a wall, within which I did not need to reveal much about myself and own feelings.

There needs to be a helpful measure of resilience alongside vulnerability. When we become too self-sufficient, we remove the possibility of help from others. We need to receive as well as to give – that is balance.

The awakening certainly had begun, yet I was to discover there was vast expansion still on the horizon.

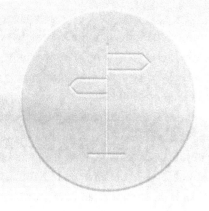

CHAPTER THREE

A reorientation

I nearly died in March 2016 and I can truly say there was no fear involved. Now in my late thirties, I embraced the requisite emergency medical treatment that was needed, from a place of acceptance and gratitude. I recovered incredibly swiftly from being on my knees with a bad flu virus, a referred bacterial infection that had culminated in chest sepsis, and renal failure of my transplant kidney. How's that for an adventure?

The years preceding this experience were ones of deep self-inquiry and looking at my life through a much more powerful lens of truth, which brought me to a place of strength and fortitude. It also presented me with the valuable opportunity to consider what my soul yearned for in this lifetime. What was I here to do? My receptive capacity to deeply question all of this was growing exponentially.

It was in Peru in Summer 2015, deep in the Andes, that the word 'dialysis' kept coming to my mind. Over and over. Whispers of it. I had to sit with that and be with it, and acknowledge why it was coming through.

I had chosen Peru to complete 500 hours of yoga training. I returned home after a month of deep, soulful inner enquiry, fascinating spiritual experiences, amazing and wholesome vegetarian food, dancing with nature and almost passing out in a sweat lodge. I felt happy to be home, but inside I was not well in a physical sense, so I started to build in a lot more rest, and avoid what felt like toxic situations and draining people. I decided to go to America after Christmas. I knew it would be my last hurrah with Kenny kidney and I had a phenomenal time. I managed to trundle on back home until March, when I caught a terrible flu after helping with my sister's kids when she and her husband were away. Both the little people had flu. My latest clinic appointment had shown a further decline to ten per cent in my kidney function and I really was not feeling at all well. I had no real reserves to draw upon, so discernment and self-preservation became key. Who you spend time with, professionally and personally, matters.

'Where are we going with this?' my renal nurse asked after she'd taken a bad blood pressure reading, and heard I had woken up that morning and been sick. Good question. All I knew was that I was exhausted, had nothing left in the tank, but was ready for what was next. Because I knew a steam train was coming right for my chest. I could feel it. That was the vision I had very clearly. And it came. Big and hard and unforgiving, and I was utterly powerless to avoid it. It was almost as if this was the catharsis into blasting through more layers and moving closer to understanding the nature of being alive. A life.

I caught the flu and self-diagnosed it as bronchitis as it went right to my chest, just as the hurtling steam train vision had shown me. I kept waking up each day and having to cancel all my obligations. My voice was barely audible. At no point did I reflect; Ciara, this is extremely serious and you need to go to the hospital. I kept waiting and seeing each day if there would be improvement. But there was none. I had no appetite, a raging headache and wasn't sleeping. It was 'bleak house,' as my sister said on coming to visit. My life force was gradually ebbing away. I had lost the ability to think sensibly and was nearly no more. Family concern was setting in. Unbeknown to me, Aisling was prepping my parents, 'Ciara is really not well'. Marley had also caught the flu so was in no state to help and Parley offered to come down, as they were getting worried. My sister and her family were going on holiday, so she was keen to ensure I was ok before they left.

Amusingly, I had previously agreed to look after my sister's dog, Ruby, while they were away. She's an extremely big hearted and enthusiastic Hungarian Vizsla, who I love. Poor Ruby, who is normally so lively, seemed to pick up on my energy levels and just sat by the lounge door like a sphinx looking outside to the garden. Every now and then she would come and sniff me lying on the sofa. I think she was checking I was still alive. The next day, once it was agreed I needed to take myself off to hospital, friends of my sister's came to pick Ruby up. I don't know why I thought I was in any state to mind her for the week. Again, another indication of just not thinking clearly as my body was effectively shutting down.

The time had come for medical intervention. Before she left for her holiday, Aisling called the out of hours GP to get me to talk to a doctor. We eventually connected and I was told an appointment was available at 1 a.m on the Saturday morning. The last thing I could face at that stage was leaving the flat and going out, alone, into the early hours. I promised my sister I would call the next day and seek advice. So she was back onto me the next morning: "Have you spoken to them?" "Yes!" I said. "I'm waiting for a call back." Ridiculously, my mobile phone was playing up and I missed the call. Argh!

Behind the scenes, the doctor trying to get hold of me was also speaking to my sister, saying, "She's not answering. If she doesn't answer, we'll have to send the police round to kick the door in."

"Please keep trying, I know she's there," she pleaded.

Thankfully, he then rang my landline and I was told exactly what I knew I needed to hear.

"This is a medical emergency given your history. Get yourself to A&E. I can send an ambulance but it'll take about four hours, so you're better off just getting yourself there now."

He said it so clearly and with such conviction, I knew it to be true as soon as I heard it.

It was a deep relief. I knew inside that it was very serious and that I needed to take action, but I needed to also lean into the support of appropriate advice. At that point on the Saturday, my sister and her family were en route to their ski holiday, so my long time good friend Vicks quickly arrived in an Uber to take me to A&E. I wonder how many Ubers now take care of medical emergencies! I remember sitting in the back of the taxi, barely able to move, very chesty and very depleted, with Vicks holding my hand and reassuring me. Even forming words was a huge effort.

We got out of the taxi and crossed the road at the lights towards the A&E entrance, me fully leaning into Vicks for support, as I could barely walk and breathing was an incredible effort.

It was a long wait, and I was so relieved to be finally seen and to be allocated a bed in the emergency department. Bloods were run and a canula inserted, ready for intravenous administration of whatever would be needed. Chest x-ray revealed chest sepsis. I was drifting in and out of a vague reality of unwellness and pain, although I remained lucid enough to be able to answer questions. I recall hearing the odd noise – a low moaning coming from a drunk Irish man. I discovered that actually, when people are very sick, they moan. I was doing it! It's a low moan, almost as if to reassure oneself or even anyone that can hear, there is a bit of life left. It's less exhausting than forming words and is deeply primal. I hear women also make this moaning sound when giving birth. Connecting to that primal instinct and deeply embedded ancestral coding.

The staff in the A&E were all brilliant. The blood chemistry came back. Creatinine 750. Urea 56. Oh God. Renal failure. It's gone. It's finished. I accepted and processed it in seconds. I brought my hands to my face and felt the beginnings of starting to cry, and then realised I did not need to. I now know it is possible, from a deep place of humility and surrender, to come away from trauma and to accept. I experienced it for myself in those few, fleeting moments. I acknowledged and I let it go. I felt so very supported by a hugely benevolent energy all around me. It was pure and unconditional love. It was utterly beautiful. I describe it as falling into the arms of trust. I felt held within a strong source of pure love.

The previous few years of declining kidney function helped me to face many fears and old stories. I spent those years deeply enquiring, helping myself as much as possible on a physical level, engaging with a deeper yoga practice, doing daily meditation, talking about it more with my own network and closest friends. I was searching for truth and connecting with the light of my soul. And, importantly, being compassionate about my own experiences. This was such a powerful realisation for me and it held me safely in this life threatening situation.

It was time to release. I sent a message of thanks to Kenny kidney. Thank you. Thank you for all the good years you gave me. Thank you for being such a precious partner in my journey in this body. Thank you for the freedom. Thank you for the wisdom. Thank you for the most beautiful of partnerships. I love you always.

The A&E doctor called the renal team. Fortunately, I was in the same hospital where my overall care is, so two doctors from the renal ward came down to see me.

"How does she look?" one of them asked Vicks.

"Well, in the 25 years I've known her, I've never seen her looking this bad," she replied.

He could tell I was dehydrated. He said the last resort was dialysis but they would do what they could. I just knew I was in the right place physically, but also mentally and emotionally, to ride this wave. I had no doubt that my recovery would be swift and remarkable. I could feel it that very night as I was transferred from A&E to the renal ward. I accepted all the treatment as it was needed. The intravenous antibiotics and the bicarb drip for the metabolic acidosis. Two strong painkillers to relieve the pounding headache, as my body struggled to stabilise temperature and homeostasis. These were the only painkillers I took, to take the edge off the horrendous headache. I needed no more.

It was late into the night and Vicks headed away once I had been safely received by the renal ward. I had my own room and was so glad to sleep. To rest. To continue the surrendering process.

I felt much improved already the next day. Of course, I was still in renal failure, but I could feel the antibiotics were getting the infection under control. Dialysis was necessary, so I had a catheter fitted into a vein in the very top of my right thigh. Not the most convenient of places and I was literally laid bare to have it inserted. I had two sessions of the blood dialysis over the next two days and it helped to bring the levels down, to clean my blood and to ease the pressure.

The official diagnosis was influenza type B, chest sepsis and renal failure. Any of these things in isolation are tough enough for the body to rebalance and heal from. All three at the same time and with a transplant kidney – phew! That's a roller-coaster ride for sure.

During the haemodialysis sessions, which were necessary to get the toxins down, I had no revisit of trauma from old memories as a teenager. I was present with the experience and the context, and was greatly relieved I wasn't triggered. This feeling of being held kept me present to what was actually happening, and stopped me from fretting about what was I to do. I had already asked all those deeper questions of myself in the previous couple of years. I got the real chance to benefit from a meaningful spiritual excavation. I had dismantled so many old stories that here I was free to heal and get well. When one is in this space, it doesn't matter what chaos is going around you, or if medical staff are being dismissive. I was just in a place of observation.

Everything was happening very quickly, as time was not on my side. Decisions need to be made swiftly in a situation like this. But I do believe it all happened in the kindest way possible. It was very serious, but necessitated quick action and compelled decisions to be made. The kidney had been on its last legs and the flu came along and knocked the remaining meaningful function out of it, so I had to decide which form of dialysis I would opt for. This is where my last clinic visit before catching the flu came into play – the one where I was feeling pretty rotten and the nurse, a straight-talking Australian who I liked and respected, had asked, "Where are we going with this?" At that time, I was still in the process of being marked up to be re-listed for another kidney, but it already seemed as if the existing kidney would not last to see me through to a second transplant. Treatment options would need to be considered to cover this period of time and to keep me well and healthy. And at that same visit, the nurse planted a powerful seed when she suggested that I'd do well on the peritoneal dialysis (PD).

"But I'd have to have a catheter," I muttered.

"You'll need that either way," she said.

Fair point. I'd asked for my fistula in my left arm, the previous haemodialyisis access site, to be tied off after my transplant when I was twenty-one, so this was no longer available as an access point. Access is a key issue in dialysis, whichever form you opt for; in fact, there are whole teams dedicated to 'access' in this renal medicine context.

As a result of that very short conversation, I felt confident to now opt for PD. This uses a glucose solution, which is moved into the abdomen through the catheter, left to dwell, and then drained out. I opted for the one where a machine runs the fluids in and out over eight hours, at night. Whilst it's long, it's more gentle than blood dialysis, and done while asleep. Essentially, it is a combination of osmosis and diffusion through the solution that works to reduce the uraemic toxins in the blood to a more manageable level.

I can't imagine I'd have found this an easy decision without that brief conversation and the huge and sudden illness coming along. It gifted me even more perspective and released me into a beautiful place of surrender and trust.

I knew in my heart the PD option felt right. Knowing my body so well, it was frankly scary to consider the insertion of an abdominal catheter, especially as a yoga teacher who is very active. However, I felt I had been guided towards this decision by a benevolent sequence of events and proceeded to have the catheter fitted. We discussed this further in light of me being a yoga teacher and petite, so a small paediatric catheter was chosen. Reassuringly, the nurse who fitted the catheter felt it would be fine to resume my own yoga practice in time. I learned they had only recently had approval to source different sizes of catheter. Up until then, it was one size for everyone. So, another great piece of timing for me.

The nurse who fitted the catheter did an excellent job. It was testament to her as a practitioner that she was trained in this surgical procedure, which allowed patients to have this done swiftly and with a local anaesthetic. In other places, I believe this is sometimes done under a general anaesthetic, which would have been an incredible strain on my body at that point.

So this led to a very quick recovery. Bearing in mind this was all only four days after being admitted in such a serious condition, and I was already feeling very much on the mend and incredibly upbeat. I utterly surrendered and felt at times I was floating on and inside clouds of love. Messages of love, support and good intention came flowing in from friends, family and colleagues. I could feel it viscerally, all this love, and felt very much supported by it. But I wasn't reliant on it as I felt such deep and quiet contentment from my very soul.

It took a couple of days for me to look at the exit site of the catheter. It had been tunnelled in just underneath the umbilicus and the exit was just to the right of my belly button. I was frankly scared to look at the reality of a tube protruding from my belly. I also noticed I was walking with a stoop due to the pain in the abdominals. I had to consciously adjust my posture upright so I could heal with an open front body. Visualisation becomes very profound in the healing process. See it in your mind's eye and so it will be. Imagination is powerful.

After the virology had been run on various swabs taken, it was confirmed I had influenza type B and was an infection risk. Due to this result the pharmacist came bouncing in, announcing he had some Tamiflu for me to take. It seemed utterly ridiculous to me that this had been prescribed and I clearly stated I would not be taking it. Instinctively, I did not want to touch that drug and practically speaking it was pointless, as I was already well out the other side of the infection. I was easily able to justify this decision, as the medication itself recommended taking it upon initial onset of symptoms, which had been many days previous. I discovered it was the virologist who had advised this course of treatment and had nothing to do with the renal team, meaning my actual main care. It's useful to be aware of who is recommending what, so you as the patient understand the context more fully for yourself.

As the hospital food was so unappealing, I really did not eat much that week – and having not been hungry the previous week at home, I was hankering for good, wholesome food by the time I was discharged. I do believe that because my system had effectively been in fasting mode for almost two weeks, this would have triggered considerable autophagy (the body's way of cleaning house), hence my progress was vastly swifter.

I was released from hospital just under a week after my admission. It was Easter weekend, so I had lots of visitors and lovely home-made food from my best friend Anna, whose Polish mother made me delicious apple cake and pancakes. I ate it all, with great relish and appreciation. My body was already very much better – now came the time to really support it and aid its healing, with lots of rest, healthy food and the love from friends and family. I told myself that I would take as much time as I needed to recover. If that meant a month or two, so be it. That's ok. However, I was able to resume my schedule after just one week of being back home. The first yoga class I taught, I went home after and slept for two hours. But I had a FIRE in my belly, a fire of hope, of gratitude, of further initiation into my sacred path. I was alive, my goodness, I was wholly alive. I know what it means now to have that sense of cracking your heart wide open to let the world fall in.

At the time all of this happened, I had already stepped away from corporate life a few years previously to set up Wholly Aligned, after spending a number of years studying nutrition and then yoga. I do believe a large part of my swift and amazing recovery stemmed from already being in a place of fulfilment; I was already doing what I loved, and felt satisfied in my heart. I'd spent about fourteen years climbing the corporate ladder before that, having many interesting and useful life experiences. This presented me with the opportunity to Wholly Align myself! To step even more into alignment with what feels true. I had spent three years studying nutrition at the excellent College of Naturopathic Medicine, at a time when I was still working full-time in banking, so it meant essentially three years of weekends were now spoken for to study and gain student clinical practise. I loved it. Yoga had always been a seed sprouting within me, as Marley trained in the 70s in South Africa for her teacher training. Yoga and nutrition go beautifully hand in hand as tools to heal and understand yourself more.

Owing largely to the deep spiritual journey of the preceding years, this episode of illness, facilitated a true recalibration. The realisation for me that I was already whole, and all that I needed resided within me. We all can benefit from remembering that. All you need is already within you.

CHAPTER FOUR

Powerful Tools: Nutrition

Let's talk about COX! Yes, you read right! I think if you understand COX, many other things will fall into place in terms of how you can best nurture your inner environment and your overall health. COX is the abbreviation for cyclo-oxygenase, also known as prostaglandins, a class of enzyme key to the inflammation pathways in the body. Non-steroidal anti-inflammatory drugs (NSAIDS), such as ibuprofen, block the action of both COX 1 and COX 2. This is damaging, as COX 1 has many protective aspects, including protecting gut tissue and kidney tissue.

This is why I do not recommend ibuprofen to anyone and encourage people who are relying on it (it's frighteningly common) to consider what's really going on, and educate themselves around options. Indeed, nephrologists are aware that these drugs are absolutely contra-indicated in kidney illness. My view is if they are damaging for at risk groups, why put them into anyone else? There are many other useful interventions, using food and mindset, which influence physiology and help with pain issues. Food influences these enzyme pathways and we can see how it nourishes or distorts the inflammatory cascade. Turmeric is a great example, as it calms inflammation without any of the highly undesirable side effects of NSAIDS.

The word diet actually stems from the Greek word dietata, which translates to 'way of life'. But look how we have distorted the term and created a hideously toxic industry around 'fat free', 'sugar free' and 'diet drinks'. None of this reflects its original meaning. Eating is part of your way of life. It consists not only of what you eat, but also how you eat, where you eat and who you eat with. This all matters and has a bearing on your digestion, metabolic rate and assimilation of nutrients.

I have always had a strong interest in food, particularly in relation to my health. I understood the link between eating well and feeling well. This grew from my very in-tune and wise doctor in South Africa, who advised minimal refined sugar, no processed foods and plenty of hydration with clean water. As I was a child, he made it more fun and interactive by asking me to draw eight glasses of water a day, one glass each time I drank it, so by the end of the day I'd have eight pencil drawn pictures of a glass, representing my water intake. And this felt entirely natural to me. I was never disbelieving or mistrustful of his advice, as he was such a kind man and had only safe wisdom to pass onto me. I often wonder now how lovely it would have been to have known him as an adult, to understand more deeply his approach and what had inspired him to practise medicine in that way. In hindsight, he certainly planted an enormous seed in me of how I wish to be with my patients. And imagine if he had stayed my doctor for longer. My wondering is very much part of inspiring hope, rather than looking back with regret and anger. I have walked through this burning fire to emerge and share this with you.

Nutrition can create powerful change within the body and the mind. Food is information to your cells. I recall one lady telling me how she had stopped drinking coffee as it had a strong depressive impact on her. Whilst it took some time to tune into the cause of her low mood, she said it was an almost instant change once the coffee drinking ceased. It is tremendously meaningful that by changing one simple thing in her routine, she alleviated a big issue in her day-to-day life. This also highlights the problem of the one size fit all approach, as many people are fine with coffee. The issue could also be the type of coffee you are drinking, so things are really never black and white. Things must always be considered in context.

A few months following my kidney transplant in 1997, Marley found a local nutritional therapist for me to see. Back in the Nineties, there was not the same wide presence of nutritional therapists as there is today. She was a kind and lovely woman. However, she had not worked with someone in my situation before. But still she approached it with an open mind, and did her best to understand the drug protocol I was on. Her recommendations involved a strict elimination diet removing wheat, red meat, sugar, alcohol and dairy. It was only for a few weeks and I'm sure this helped calm systemic inflammation in the body. It also served as a reminder to take care of myself. It's good to rest the body from heaviness without needing to commit to a lifetime of eating in this way, especially when it is in a potent recovery phase.

The first liver cleanse I ever did in my late twenties; I distinctly remember going to a yoga class the day after finishing it and being amazed at how clean my muscles felt. It was a new sensation and it felt vey good. I was still taking immune-suppression medication, so arguably it was not the best time to have done it, but at that time I had not trained in nutrition or yoga and was exploring ways to help myself feel better. It was a five day cleanse, where I ate only fruit and vegetables on days one and five, and fasted on herbal teas and a vegetable broth to support the liver on the middle three days . The first couple of days were tough and plenty of rest was needed to support the cleanse. At times it felt almost like a flu was coming on.

This revealed to me how much the body will put up with. When we give it space and nourishment to recalibrate, it can be fascinating what literally gets pulled out of your tissues.

Nutrition is a deeply personal thing. It is, after all, how we nourish ourselves, our bodies and our minds, but it can also be how we sabotage our existence. When I turned 30, I really began to dive deeper into the relationship I had with alcohol. In a modern and especially western society, alcohol is so widely socially accepted, often in quite dangerous quantities. This makes it all the more pernicious, especially when people are conditioned to believe that drinking is fun.

Given my constitution I never had a large capacity for booze, which I certainly took some time to be honest with myself about. Yes, I have been too inebriated on occasion in younger years and from that made quite unwise choices. It was often a lot of fun to cut loose in that way, but there comes a point when we need to reflect on our patterns, and consider if they are truly serving us. This requires guts and courage. It's not easy to break addictive patterns. But it is entirely possible and so that is where it helps to remain hopeful.

I drink very little alcohol these days. I also have found the more one tunes into noticing the effects things might be having, the less inclined one is to be tempted. It becomes far less interesting and, indeed, the body becomes far more sensitive to it. Alcohol is a huge driver of disease in our society. After I'd had the kidney transplant, I regularly suffered from dreadful migraines, and alcohol and stress were certainly triggers for these. The cyclosporin immune-suppression drug I was taking also depleted my magnesium levels, which could have been a contributing factor to the migraines. They were a useful way, I now realise, to force me to slow down. With these migraines all I could do was lie in a dark room until it passed. The body will tell you what it needs. If rest is needed, your body will tell you again – and again – until you listen and respond. This is one of the reasons self-care is so utterly key. We revolutionise humanity through the action of loving self-care.

My toe inflammation was subsequently diagnosed as pseudo gout, so called as my uric acid levels were not elevated as they are in traditional gout. I really did not wish to have recurrence of it, as it was such a painful experience. Again, I looked at ways to help myself, including nourishing my emotions as it felt like this was a big aspect to the physical presentation. The more overall physical, emotional and mental work I did, the more my body was able to lift itself out of these experiences. I'm delighted to say I have had no further recurrence of these and feel it's now been released from my body. I never took any medication for this when it recurred, as the side effects on the kidneys were not good. Instead, I discovered that resting with the affected body part elevated helped, along with specific dietary additions. This included celery juice and celery, along with cherries or a pure form of cherry juice, and staying well hydrated to flush it out. Limiting rich foods such as meat, dairy and alcohol was also helpful whilst the body was working to clear the issue. In addition, I found the regular application of black pepper essential oil very useful: diluting two to three drops in a base oil and rubbing it into the toe area. Bathing the affected area with a good splash of unfiltered apple cider vinegar helped too. So instead of taking a pill that is likely to damage other parts of your body, explore how you can support your body towards healing, using its innate wisdom.

What works for you can also change throughout your life. As adults we've moved on from suckling at our mother's breast. We transition through different life stages and thus our nutritional requirements change. A renal nurse once said to me, "There's no such thing as a renal diet." It was a comment made as part of a wider nutrition/lifestyle discussion, but that particular remark landed with me. Of course there's no such thing as a renal diet. All 'kidney patients' are advised on certain dietary considerations. However, all will eat according to their existing cultural patterns. For example, a 50 year old Indian man who eats a traditional Indian diet, will eat entirely differently to a teenage girl following a vegetarian diet, even though both might be kidney patients. This is a really important point, as I often see renal patients getting very fixated on limiting things and missing the bigger picture. In particular, I see this on the online Health Unlocked community I run, where I post about yoga and nutrition. I set this up after I stopped holding onto a lot of the emotional charge from my health experience, and being able to share from a place of practical counsel is great. Before, I would get too triggered by other renal patients. I see people on the kidney forums get very panicked about being diagnosed whilst their kidney function still remains very good. My view is there is much upside to be had from a holistic approach to understanding one's body and mind connection. If we get fixated on what not to eat, it pushes panic and fear deeper into the tissues. Instead, take the pedal off the panic button and ease into honesty and self-compassion, and from that place explore what you can change. Let the chapter on the wellbeing fund help you with this. All of it matters. It's always all about the context and only you can know your own context.

Let me give you an example of this context. I remember being ravenous after the evening dialysis sessions as a teenager. As Parley knew I would be hungry, he would make me a sandwich so it was ready for me when we got home.

There it would be sitting on the kitchen table, with a piece of kitchen towel thoughtfully draped over it. And I would sit down and eat it with great joy. Now, that was my context, because I would not usually advise people to be eating late night sandwiches. However, that is what I needed during that phase, as I would have been going straight from school to the session without supper. Very occasionally, he might not have the chance to make me a sandwich and I would be crestfallen to come home to an empty kitchen table. "Where's my sandwich?!" I might have roared, a bit like Ross from Friends in the episode where his boss eats the sandwich his sister has made him. He needed to be tranquilised, he was so upset about it! I sympathise! Whenever I watch that episode it makes me laugh a lot. This story also perhaps explains the strong association of comfort I get from bread. I have gone through various stages of eliminating it, but my soul always yearns for its return. So, as part of being kind to myself, I have it when I feel like having it. It represents to me the love and kindness of my father, who uncomplainingly drove me home from late night dialysis.

Typically, I choose a bread that is a good quality sourdough, rather than supermarket bread, and it continues to be a food that brings me overall nourishment. Some breads will make me feel inflamed and unwell in my joints, but this is mostly due to the fast acting yeast, or other unknown additives. It tends not to happen with home baked soda bread or a good sourdough, neither of which have any commercial yeast or flour improvers. Organic flour is also a significant component, as when grains are not grown or stored organically they are exposed to all manner of pesticides and fungicides.

I have at times been caught up in the obsession our society now has with cutting things out, but have not found it to be helpful as it's easy to become fixated. I absolutely advocate short term adjustments, so eliminating something for a few weeks, for example, and seeing how you feel can be good. But be ready. When we 100 per cent commit to an endeavour, we succeed. If we half-heartedly say we are going to cut something out, like wheat or sugar or alcohol, if we have not internally committed, it's not going to work. Readiness is key.

You need to decide what works for you, but in my experience being too restrictive tends to bring mental fixations. So when I tell my brain I can have what I like, I am more balanced and in turn the likelihood of rebound eating and poor choices is reduced. And the more we enhance the health of our own inner forest – our gut biome – the more the body and mind thrives. What we eat and drink does have an impact on mood – think

about a punishing hangover! What we put in matters, as does our ability
to process it safely without creating bundles of metabolic endotoxins,
which are increasingly coming up as the key driver of many disease
processes. An endotoxin means it is something metabolised internally so,
for example, the metabolic waste from food digestion. When we have a
robust gut biome, these endotoxins tend to be less problematic. When
we do not, and many ongoing factors will influence that, the result can be
oxidation leading to cellular inflammation. The studies on this from just
one particular fast food meal shows massive effect on increased levels of
endotoxins in the blood. Research microbiologist, Kiran Krishnan, who
speaks brilliantly on the microbiome and who conducted the research
study, has created a spore probiotic (unfortunately not suitable for organ
transplant recipients) that is helping with metabolic endotoxemia.

Digestion is a complex process and it begins the moment we smell or
even think of food. This speaks to the importance of artful preparation. We
stimulate the salivary glands and digestive juices as we chop up the herbs
and garlic and breathe in the aromas. This first step is now often left out,
as we eat more processed, ready-made food in a rushed state. A digestion
disaster! In Ayurveda, the traditional Indian wisdom system of health,
often a slice of ginger with lime juice and a tiny pinch of sea salt is eaten
before a meal to encourage the digestive juices. Very important! We must
switch on our juices in order to promote healthy and effective digestion.
Think of it as food foreplay!

Eating in a crammed state does not facilitate healthy digestion. We are
tipped into a sympathetic nervous system state, known as 'fight or flight,'
or survival mode. We are not designed to eat in this way. Eating in a
tranquil, contented state is vital. This plays into the social relevance of food
and how food brings us together. We cook and create with love for the
ones we care for. We share in the delicious aromas. This moves us safely
into 'rest and digest' mode, where the para-sympathetic nervous system

can switch on. And we need to be able to move effortlessly and smoothly between these states of being.

Unfortunately, what is happening on a massive scale is 'hyper survival,' as I call it. We are revved up creating high adrenaline and cortisol levels. The more we are in survival mode, the more we stay there. The pattern becomes set as the body feels in a perpetual state of alarm. At risk. On standby for attack. Therefore, the slightest stress will create an over-response. It becomes a very dangerous spiral, leaving us marinating in a soup of stress hormones, which comes out in anger, poor immunity, inflammation, hyper-tension and fast heartbeat, to name but a few. These patterns are a key driver in the pervasive chronic disease we see across our supposed civilised world. And on top of all that, the general acceptance of reaching for very damaging painkillers is of concern. How far are we removed from feeling pain? We cannot numb ourselves to this extent. That is not nourishment. Consider if your adrenal glands are hats of hope on top of your kidneys, or hats of fear. I feel this ties in very well with the view in Traditional Chinese Medicine that the emotion of fear is related to kidneys.

When I worked in banking in a very hectic Canary Wharf in London, you could easily be swallowed up and never see daylight, just screens and artificial lighting. From the tube train commute to your desk, to the canteen, to the gym after work. All set up to keep you near your desk, to keep you in the office. They started to sell postage stamps in the coffee shop on the ground floor – might seem a considered convenience – but I saw this as just one more way to keep us from needing to go outside. And the ramifications of such a lifestyle is showing up all over the place now. Awareness is spreading and open minded companies are investing in the promotion of health much more. There is a long way to go, but the shift is definitely there.

We all oscillate between patterns. Where it gets tricky is when patterns bed down and you find yourself needing a glass of wine every night to be able to cope with your day. The presence of alcohol in our western society is too widely accepted and over consumed. I certainly went through phases where I drank too much, in the context of what was right for me. The ability to relax and self soothe gets annihilated and this is where addiction can begin to take hold: be it sex, alcohol, caffeine, sugar or cocaine. These patterns need to be acknowledged in order to be broken. Addiction, at its bare bones, is a lack of self-love. We cannot numb the pain as we drive it deeper. Pain is a way your body is communicating to you. Listen to it. Think about what is ultimately driving this pain. Deep seated emotional pain does get stuck.

A little planning goes a long way. Shop consciously. Do not underestimate the power you have as a paying consumer. Support shops that stock local, seasonal and organic as much as possible. It's important and, collectively, we can absolutely make a difference. Does it mean you must become puritanical and obsessive about what and how you eat? No! It defeats the purpose of healthy eating if it becomes a strain and riddled with anxiety. If you fancy a piece of cake have it – and, importantly, enjoy it. It's all about balance and what works for you, and makes you feel well. But better to have a home baked cake than a factory packet one that is likely to be full of hydrogenated oils and too much sugar. The energetics of food matters. A meal lovingly prepared by yourself or a loved one carries so much more nourishment than one made commercially.

I watched an interesting food documentary some years ago. One scene that stuck with me was filmed in Las Vegas, where they showed huge trucks pumping tons of fatty muck into massive holes that had been dug way out in the desert. Where was this muck from? The drains of Las Vegas, reflecting the amount of dangerous hydrogenated fats the multiple fast food restaurants produced. It blocked up the drains, and the big trucks had to come and pump it out and dispose of it on desert land. To me this was very symbolic of what we are doing to our own bodies. Eating too much, eating in a rush, eating in a bad mood and clogging up our own intricate cardiovascular systems. The microcosm is a reflection of the macrocosm, meaning our bodies are a reflection of the wider universe. Our guts are a reflection of the wider ecosystem. Deforestation happening on a mass global scale is also indicative of what is happening in our own inner ecosystem of the microbiome. All is connected.

For us, the big trucks are the over worked NHS coming in and attempting to unclog and mop up the damage. But all that muck has to go somewhere, because the root cause of all of this is not being addressed at a sufficiently wide, national or global level. Imagine the doctors who now have to regularly saw off feet and legs as a result of unmanaged diabetes. How distressing must that be for them – that's a horrific part to play. How could it get to the stage that someone needs an amputation? How have we created a society where people truly are lost on how to nourish themselves well? There is no need for this. We now have evidence that type 2 diabetes can be reversible through diet and lifestyle changes. Putting synthetic insulin into a body that is burned through dietary and lifestyle habits is disastrous. Dr Jason Fung, Toronto based nephrologist, is doing marvellous work in this arena. Everyone has their message to share and you can simply find what you need.

And so, we start with ourselves. We start slowly, especially if we have not had the foundation of good nutrition as children. It's never too late to learn new, healthful habits and make improved choices. Start with boiling an egg, start somewhere. This is a huge step towards taking responsibility and enjoying your food.

Food is information for our cells to signal and respond to. It influences our gene expression and DNA methylation pathways. So if anyone tells you that what you eat has no bearing on your health, ring the alarm bell! Spot when bullshit is bullshit and truth is truth. You can do this by opening up truly to your own inner physician. It's there! Connect with it. Trust your intuitive response to situations more, including the foods you take into your body.

I work with people on the basis they are a unique and individual person, and one size does not fit all when it comes to food. What I do advocate is eating real food and moving your body in ways that is enjoyable to you. Wholesome food and physical movement are two cornerstones to a healthy body and mind, another being sleep. This does not translate to deprivation. I love coffee and drink a black coffee every morning. Although in the past I have given it up, it's a struggle to stop, and I get a lot of enjoyment from it. It's one a day and with food, so it is not an intense blood sugar/cortisol and adrenaline spike, which happens when drinking coffee on its own, especially first thing in the morning on an empty stomach. You can make a change by switching to starting with hot water and lemon and then have your coffee with your breakfast. Our cortisol levels peak around 8 am as the body prepares to be energised for the day, so having a coffee around that time is better, as it then avoids cortisol spiking outside its rhythm later in the day.

Getting good quality sleep, being well hydrated, and eating a nutrient dense diet are general tips that are relevant to most people. Understand yourself and listen to your own body. Be the wisest physician you know for yourself. Deeply enquire within, so you can deeply respond and let that response power and motivate conscious change in your patterns, to help you thrive. From this place, advice that you seek will be more helpful and you will be able to see more clearly.

What do I do in terms of nourishing myself? I listen to the needs of my body as much as possible. For me, rest is a key part of my wellness and I have about nine hours sleep a night. The current dialysis treatment I need is eight hours, six nights a week, so I know I need at least that amount of sleep, especially if I have a disturbed night with the machine alarming, or the drain causing me pain.

More and more, I eat home cooked food. When I do eat out, I choose places I trust as much as possible - that have an honest and enthusiastic approach to food. I always start the day with a large mug of boiled water with half a lemon squeezed into it. On days I accidentally run out of lemons, I really miss that morning zing. I stay well hydrated with filtered water. Although I do eat bread, I only eat pasta, rice or potatoes on occasion. Organic sourdough bread is a strong recommendation from me as it is made in the traditional, slow rise manner with no nasty, commercial fast acting yeast which, in my opinion, can add a great burden to the digestive system. There are, of course, cases where gluten is truly a problem. Marley, for example, does not tolerate it well. If gluten makes you feel unwell this can manifest in many ways, such as swollen joints and general low mood, as well as the more obvious digestive complaints such as abdominal pain, bloating and excessive gas, along with foul smelling stools. You might find you eliminate it for a few months and are able to introduce it back. The other issue with wheat is when it is commercially grown, harvested and stored, it is exposed to pesticides. Some grains can be stored for up to two years, so the risk of mould and insect infestation is quite high. In organic farming, the grains are not subjected to these chemicals. So, likely one of the other reasons that wheat has become so challenging to digest is that today's processes are far removed from how it was first grown and harvested. This is why I encourage people to invest in organic foods as much as possible. Does it have to be organic every single time? No. Take a view on what works for you and do your own research.

Keep checking in with yourself to make sure you are not getting too fixated. Your path needs to be a balance between challenge and nourishment – the middle path, as Buddhists encourage. Or a little of what you fancy, as Marley says.

It is heartening to see the big shift currently happening in the world of medicine and food. We have strong figures within the medical community, such as Dr Jason Fung and Dr Rangan Chatterjee, who are true activists and sharing from a place of experience. That they both trained as nephrologists makes them more interesting to me personally! There is also an increasing amount of literature on the benefits of fasting to the body. As mentioned, in the run up to my hospital episode in 2016, I essentially fasted for the whole week before, as I was so ill and had zero appetite. It's likely this triggered substantial autophagy, which happens when we fast and is the body's clever way of cleaning house. I do feel instinctively that this contributed to my swift recovery. I barely ate the week I was in hospital. It may well be that as my system was open and without food to digest and assimilate, the intravenous antibiotics I received worked more effectively. They kicked in so quick, in a matter of hours, to bring down a considerable state of sepsis and systemic inflammation. I also realised it had been an inherent pattern of mine to include long periods of fasting throughout my life. I remember my brother-in-law saying to me many years ago: "I know now why you are so slim, because sometimes you eat a lot and then you'll have periods when you eat not much." Each day is different, so just keep tuning in.

It is also useful to be aware of what medications might be contributing to certain nutrient depletions. This is where understanding pharmacology for yourself is very relevant. For example, cyclosporin, which was the main immuno-suppression drug I took for many years, depletes both Vitamin C and magnesium. This is important information and no medical professional or pharmacist vocalised this clearly to me – although it is buried in the reams of side effects that comes with these medications. I also wonder how this information on side effects is gathered, as over the years I have never knowingly been asked about this. I wonder, is it all anecdotal, or just based on small and limited, pharmaceutically funded research?

Both Vitamin C and magnesium play considerable roles in our body. So, in some cases supplementation might be necessary, depending on the severity of your symptoms. But, of course, dietary intervention is the safest 'supplementation' of all. Eat plenty of magnesium rich foods, swim in the sea and bathe in epsom salts (epsom salts are just pure magnesium in its sulphate form). Those are some ways of getting your magnesium and ensuring your tissues are replenished. Blood serum levels of magnesium tell very little about your overall magnesium status, so again this is where looking at the case of a patient intelligently and intuitively is very important. Muscle twitches, compromised sleep, low mood, headaches and migraines can all be indications of a low magnesium status. The other way of looking at it is to make choices that avoid the depletion of this mineral in your body. Coffee, alcohol and an overactive stress response all deplete levels of magnesium, alongside the medication. Be aware too, that any medication will be an increased burden on your liver. I shudder when I look back at my 21-year-old self after my transplant when, because of my age and new found sense of freedom, I drank too much alcohol. I used to have dreadful hangovers, in some part due to the cocktail of medications I had been taking. Although I did leave it some time post-operation before drinking, I wish I had the knowledge I have now. But I also recognise I did need to let my hair down and be wild. As Parley says, "The body is very forgiving." And that is very true. It will put up with a lot before it says, listen, enough!

And our ego needs to be sufficiently in check to hear that message! The ego, by nature, is very fear based. We have evolved through the negative bias and survivalist nature of our reptilian brains. And we dumb ourselves down hugely by eating packet dinners in front of the television. We may as well announce to the world we are there to be conditioned and programmed, in whatever way fits. We must empower ourselves to reconnect with our true nature, and eating well is very much a part of this. This is one of the reasons it feels so good to cook a nourishing meal for the people who we love and care about. There is such union that comes from eating good food together. Does this mean never eat cake? Absolutely not! A little of what you fancy, from a place of awareness. Your body will tell you what feels right. Trust, trust, trust.

Vitamin C is possibly one of the most widely researched vitamins. Some of its highest concentrations are found in the adrenal glands and the more cortisol made by the body, the more vitamin C is used up[*]. So, if you are not getting enough and are making poor lifestyle choices - such as too much caffeine and alcohol, and you have an over-excited stress response - your immunity can be compromised. Transplant patients are told their immune systems will be dampened down due to the drugs, without the bigger picture being explained. Yes, on a white blood cellular level the drugs are lowering the immunity, but we can counter some of that by ensuring we have adequate intakes of key nutrients.

I had a lovely chat with an old Irish man on the bus one day. I noticed he was a wiry, strong, muscly man although in his 70s. He said he was one of twelve and that his mother probably never had any peace. He was a carpenter by trade, which explained his physique, and he told me lovely stories about how his mother would say to him, "Now, I need twelve trout for supper please," and off he'd go to fish for them. They would pick turnips from the earth on their way home from school and eat them like apples. It was such a welcome exchange. I reflected upon this conversation and thought how powerful it would be for the nutrition movement to have people like him go and chat to schools. No confusing pseudo-science, no hidden agenda to push supplements, just tales of honest food being eaten from the sacred land. My best friend Anna tells me she used to love onion sandwiches in Poland, where she grew up. These beautiful, fresh, sweet onions from her grandmother, on proper Polish rye bread. Imagine offering an onion sandwich to a child these days? They'd tell you to eff off!

The supplement industry is huge and it's very easy for people to get lost in the choices and the advertising information. I am extremely discerning when it comes to supplements, as it's an area often not well understood by both the public and, to some extent, practitioners. I have, over the

---

[*]The American Journal of Clinical Nutrition Volume 86, Issue 1, 1 July 2007, Pages 145–149

years, come to realise there are ethical and discerning companies out there, making high quality, safe products. But many brands make their products with non-nutritive excipients, binders and fillers, which can inhibit their absorption, and there is questionable merit including them for oral ingestion. Mostly, these are added in order to make the manufacturing process easier and faster. Companies that I use, such as Premier Research in the US and Terranova here in the UK, are great companies that care what goes into their products. Pay attention to the quality of your supplements. Ideally, these should only be used during a therapeutic window to assist the body in recalibrating, whilst it heals. This is an individual timeframe, depending on the person and their ailments, and medical history. For example, if they have a Vitamin D deficiency and gut assimilation issues, prescribing certain Vitamin D supplements might be a waste of their investment, and they might need a sub-lingual form of Vitamin D instead. Or they might be better served taking pure aloe vera over a period of time, to help heal the gut tissue. These situations are multi-factorial and this links back to your physician or practitioner needing to take a good case history. They need to be tuned in and knowledgeable enough to truly help you. To meet you where you are at, both honestly and safely.

For anyone following nutrition closely, you will know the increasing evidence of fat being our friend and sugar being the enemy. That is quite a basic way of looking at this, and again it's important to consider your own needs and what suits you. However, we now know how the low fat movement, and the misinformation given by the parts of the food industry to the public, was extremely damaging. It takes a patient person, even these days, to sift though all the conflicting - and often unsubstantiated - health advice. We need good fats to be healthy. Interestingly, we also have different kinds of adipose (fat) tissue in the body. There is visceral fat surrounding our organs, subcutaneous fat just beneath the skin, and we have what's called both white and brown fat. Brown fat is sometimes referred to as good fat tissue, as its main function is to convert food into heat energy. If we look to understanding why brown fat is brown, this helps us understand why this type of fat tissue is considered better. It is brown because of plentiful mitochondria, our energy powerhouse cells, which are rich in iron. It is this that makes the fat brown. In obesity, it is mostly white fat that is present, as it seems to be the type that gets stored from excessive calories. In newborn babies, brown fat is high, which is why they don't typically shiver from the cold. Holding a new baby is a bit like hugging a hot water bottle! They are toasty warm, wrapped in brown fat and generating plentiful heat as a result.

Steps to limit availability of low nutrient and high sugar foods must be taken as part of a company's corporate responsibility. How many people work in an office where there is a coffee machine, and a vending machine full of processed sugary snacks or fizzy drinks? How did this become acceptable, and who benefits from the mass presence of these machines? For many, sugar is a deep seated addiction and this definitely shows in office life, where packets of cakes and biscuits are plentiful. Life can be naturally sweet enough. When we tune into that, we no longer need to reach for these surges of processed and damaging sweetness. One day at the bank, a colleague brought in a bin full of apples from his own garden and put them by the vending machine. It was one of those big black bins, filled with about two hundred apples. They were gone in a day. People loved them. It shows that, given good choices, people will take them. And the person who brought them benefitted too, knowing his apples were enjoyed - with no exchange of money, or plastic wrapping to be seen!

I love the approach of Dr Jason Fung, as I was heartened to find a nephrologist in the public domain speaking a lot of good sense around food. He says that it's not that helpful to focus on the macronutrients, namely high fat/low carb, or vice versa, but that it's much more the issue of people eating too many processed foods. That is the clear correlation that drives the obesity and diabetes epidemic. Drop the reliance on packet and processed foods and things will improve significantly.

I brought my own food, in case the offering was not great for the residence PD training I had to do, before getting the machine home to use on my own. I was glad I did as the kitchen was full of mostly packet, processed foods, sugary breakfast cereals and an alarmingly plentiful supply of fizzy drinks and crisps. And all of this was on offer for free. Again, how did this happen? Why are the NHS dieticians not looking at this? Much of this food is damaging to renal function and not appropriate for people whose kidneys have already been severely impaired. Fizzy pop strips the bones of calcium as the body strives to neutralise the onslaught of phosphoric acid and acid forming sugar – bone disease is an associated complication in renal impairment. These things are extremely bad for the average healthy person; putting it in front of kidney compromised patients, many of whom are also diabetic, is clearly worrying. The residential venue for the training was very pleasant and had a fully equipped kitchen, so there was no reason why fresh foods could not have been available for the patients to prepare.

I did not see a dietician through the NHS in the 17 years I was in London, and I don't recall seeing one when I had my transplant. I don't know if there is a protocol for the required amount of time a transplant patient would be seeing one and, like many protocols, this probably varies widely. There is no Gold Standard. However, on commencing PD, there was a requirement for me to see the dietician every six months. Another benefit of this form of treatment was that there were no real restrictions in terms of food choice and fluid. This made a huge difference after my seven years of haemodialysis, which was much more restrictive. I also have developed a great awareness of what works for me. I've found potassium intake is much less of an issue on this form of dialysis, based on how I metabolise potassium. I know this from watching my levels myself. I ensure I eat plenty of fibre (important with a catheter, as constipation can impact its efficacy) and whole foods and drink plenty of water. And I am able to include lots of fruits and vegetables, as my potassium stays within a safe range. I also have occasional alcohol and enjoy the odd piece of cake. I will go for days without refined sugars and usually feel much better for it.

Sugar is a big driver of inflammation, which can lead to general disease in the body. That doesn't mean eat no sugar ever. Just consider how much you might be consuming and how that is working for you. Standard protocol for all PD patients is to take a selection of up to three different laxatives. I was very clear that my intuition was telling me these were not necessary for me. So I do not take any and manage healthy bowel movements through plentiful fibre, yoga, walking, deep breathing and good hydration. Long term laxative use weakens the natural peristaltic action of the bowel muscle and I would also question what they are doing to the gut flora.

For those with kidney issues, secondary heart complications can be common. Having this knowledge empowers you to make good heart choices for yourself. One thing I have regularly is green tea. Its antioxidant profile is a good choice of regular beverage to protect the heart, as well as the bones – another important consideration in compromised kidney function. This further affirms the importance of maintaining a healthy blood pressure. I go through phases with my blood pressure. I have noticed that when my haemoglobin (Hb) levels are low, my blood pressure increases, and there is a correlation between lower Hb and an increased vasoconstriction. Managing your stress response is also absolutely relevant, as this can drive up blood pressure and heart rate – and, indeed, potentially inflammatory markers, like homocysteine and CRP. Inflamed and angry thoughts can trigger inflamed and angry tissues. Everything's connected. Your inner mental realm matters when it comes to heart health. Get good sleep and minimise the time you watch television. Through all of this, you can begin to engage more in all the variables that could be influencing how you feel, and nourish yourself.

Top tips for nutrition as your medicine

- Make one change today and let it be easy and simple. Start your day with hot water and lemon. Make a large mug boiled from the kettle and leave to cool, adding in the juice of a fresh lemon – you decide how much. Mostly, I use half a lemon. Have as the first drink of your day before food as a hydration boost and a song for your liver.

- Understand and experience the benefit of ritual when it comes to taking in food and drink. Take time to be present with what you take into your body. When you slow down, you become more present and aware of how your choices serve or sabotage you. Enjoying a delicious glass of wine with a dear friend, in a relaxed environment and deep conversation, is so much better than several glasses of wine in an awkward social setting with people you don't particularly like. What feels better? What situation will your body and mind respond more favourably to?

- If you do drink alcohol, particularly if you drink regularly and are getting hangovers, begin to examine your relationship with alcohol. I started this process when I was 30, as I started to find hangovers so deeply unpleasant – not just physically, but in terms of how it would impact my mood. Urgh! And ask yourself, am I medicating through alcohol? Why do I drink? Keep digging into the answers. I was fortunate in that I had a strong drive to eliminate toxic patterns due to my kidney condition. Find your inner motivation. Move towards balance and honesty. And be kind to yourself in the process.

- Look into getting professional nutrition advice, if you feel that is helpful to you. Find a holistic practitioner who can understand your needs. This can really help set you into a healthier rhythm and to see yourself clearly through another's eyes. If you have a specific health condition, it can be helpful to seek out a practitioner who specialises in that same thing, so they have experience of it. But, most importantly, work with someone you like and trust.

- Say farewell to ultra-processed foods, especially if you have kidney issues. Such foods are not only of very limited nutritional benefit, they are also damaging due to their increasingly chemicalised nature, and are high in phosphoric acid.

- Avoid, avoid, avoid any packet food with the ingredients of trans fats – typically labelled as hydrogenated or partially hydrogenated. These are already banned in Denmark. Well done the Danes! Why are they still in our food chain when they are one of the most toxic things to digest and a big driver to metabolic endotoxemia? Come to understand ingredients if you are buying packet food.

- Fall in love with your kitchen and get inspired to cook. Care enough to cook for yourself and your loved ones. Food made with love tastes so much better than a shop bought microwave dinner. And stay away from microwaves! It changes the DNA structure of the food that has been microwaved.

- Really examine your intake of refined and processed sugars. This is key for everyone, but especially if you are diabetic or have any issues with insulin resistance. Check food labels if you are buying anything in a packet, including basic commodities such as bread. There are plenty of resources out there to help you look more closely at this. Fizzy pop and having sugar in tea and coffee are two ways that mount up your sugar intake and, of course, beer and wine. Educate your children around this too. They are relying on you to guide them. Saying 'No' is ok and explain to them why, so they understand.

- Eat plentiful colourful fruit and vegetables, including fresh herbs such as coriander and flat leaf parsley.

- Bread – either bake your own or purchase from a trusted source e.g. a local bakery that uses ethical and organic ingredients and, ideally, a properly fermented yeast. Aim not to eat bread everyday. Variety is useful.

- Take your time when you eat. Engage with this human need for nourishment. Chew your food, slow down. Avoid eating at a desk or in front of the television. Take a moment to offer up gratitude to the earth for the food you eat. Blessing your food in a way that resonates with you is very powerful. Through that we acknowledge how fortunate we are to be fed.

- Include daily fasting windows of a minimum of 12 hours and increase this to around 16 hours when you can, perhaps twice weekly. This is helpful to trigger autophagy – the body's clever way of cleaning house. I like to think of autophagy as the Pacman effect. I loved Pacman machines as a child. Pacman is your autophagy process, munching up unhelpful cells through phagocytosis. It's great to visually imagine unhelpful cells being munched up. Nom, nom, nom.

- Look at supplement ingredients. The wonder of the nutrition found in our natural food is that the presence of vitamins and minerals work in concert, synergistically. When we supplement, this can be distorted. Supplements are therefore best taken in the right context for you, and for the optimum therapeutic window, not on an open-ended basis, unless specifically appropriate for you.

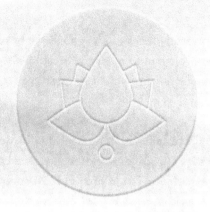

CHAPTER FIVE

Powerful Tools: Yoga and Shamanic Wisdom

Our bodies are a map for all our experiences: our fears, injuries, broken bones, broken hearts. They hold our stories. As each day brings with it opportunities for new experiences, finding a way to release the old, especially if they are holding you back, is important. Healing happens beyond the stories of the mind, meaning beyond the conditioned beliefs you have cultivated. These beliefs are set in early childhood. It's no-one's fault, as child rearing comes with challenge and parents are doing their best. However, once we reach adulthood, we are responsible for our own happiness and health. This is what I call to 'Go Beyond'. To go beyond these conditioned beliefs, we need to realise firstly that they are there, and then dismantle them. So how can we Go Beyond?

One of the most powerful processes I have found to be of great help, is to look after the body through movement and breath. This sounds incredibly simple, but truly embodying our physical experience requires learning through practise.

And it is not an intellectual pursuit, it is one that is felt deeply in our tissues. After all, our bodies are our storehouses, the maps and libraries of all we have and ever will experience. That is profound. Discovering ways to nurture the truth of our own anatomy is so helpful. I'd love to share with you what I have found helpful, and inspire you to explore your own breath and physical form. Consider what it is that moves you, literally and metaphorically. To be in alignment in body and mind. To be in alignment with your values and desires. But to do this, sometimes we need to get out of our own way. That old adage of 'you gotta lose yourself to find yourself'.

I had the gift of an early introduction to yoga, as Marley trained in the 1970s in South Africa for her yoga teacher qualification. She practised yoga during her pregnancy with me and taught children's classes at our house, so I was introduced to it from a young age. Although I enjoyed yoga as a child, when you're that age, the spiritual side of the practise is not so obvious – nor in fact necessary, as we are less bogged down by mental nonsense. I was into my late twenties when I re-connected with the practise in a fuller sense. My best friend Anna told me about the yoga class she was going to at the gym at work and suggested I give it a go. And so began my re-kindling. It was physically tough, but very quickly I began to feel stronger and started to recognise the mental benefits. This was at a time when I was working in banking in hectic Canary Wharf, so yoga also became a soothing antidote to the stress of the day.

I would go to this class twice a week. It was a reconnection that happened at a time when I was recovering from the demise of a significant five-year relationship, which had left me heartbroken. I'd practiced very little yoga during this relationship, nor did I really enjoy playing my guitar or singing. Even though I loved this man hugely, it had completely stifled me creatively and I had become blocked on many levels. The relationship, which ended four months before our wedding, took years to recover from. Losing someone you have had such deep love for, so much that you have committed to marriage, is painfully difficult. But, as always, these situations provide the catalyst for healing if we choose, and if we can see it that way. I was still emotionally very fragile and wounded from all the turmoil I had experienced with my health. As a result, I kept repeating patterns where I was attracted to men I saw as needing rescuing, missing the very fact I desperately needed to rescue myself. As such, I went on to attract a lot of dysfunctional encounters, because within myself I had not truly reflected on what a true partnership might feel like. And that I deserved to be supported as much as I supported others. I learned I must reveal myself, fully. This is not easy! It's still a work in progress, as it is for us all. But my, it's worthwhile work. I discovered there is no value in remaining hidden.

Yoga, music and songwriting came back into my life significantly when I let go of that relationship. The beauty of yoga, I feel, is what a giving practise it is. Stemming from such an ancient lineage and wisdom, it has the depth to help the practitioner move through their life stages. The body is always changing. Cells grow and die off. Circumstances change. The information we give our bodies, through food, emotions and thoughts, changes. There will always be some aspect of yoga that is right for you.

In 2009 when I was 32, I was on a beach in the Perhentian Islands off Malaysia, when I said to my friend Caroline, "I'm going to do my yoga teacher training." It took another few years to manifest that planted seed and, in 2012, I went to Andalucia in Spain, for one month, to complete a 200-hours training course to become a certified instructor. This was led by Vidya Heisel and the main focus was on vinyasa flow yoga. I love to dance and flow yoga felt like a graceful and magical dance with spirit. The yoga school was on an old converted olive farm. It was an enriching month. It was also a time when my transplant kidney flourished and I was on no pharmaceutical medications. On the surface, all was well, but my inner turbulence had still not been fully felt. This is where I have come to understand more how key it is that we feel our feelings and allow ourselves to be seen by the people closest to us. This really became a deep period of reflection and understanding of how life opens up more fully when we trust our intuition more. After this training I would be returning home to start a 3 day working week at the bank, having been offered part time when I resigned. This month provided that transition into really birthing Wholly Aligned into the world and to honouring my purpose.

Yoga cultivates consistency, regardless of the circumstances. This was a great insight from Vidya, which I found so simple and true. Attaining this when the external circumstances are changing, from joyful and elating to deeply painful and harrowing, means we have the capacity and resilience within to remain consistent within the mental realm. This doesn't mean we deny our feelings. Instead, we start to acknowledge emotions instead of suppressing, or turning away, from them. We are empowered. It is the ultimate mastery of the mind that brings us home into our hearts.

Returning from the yoga training in Spain, I discovered a whole new world of yoga happening right on my doorstep in London. I heard about a lovely studio called Indaba, and reaped tremendous benefit from attending a number of yoga workshops there. This challenged me physically and mentally, especially at a time when I was feeling very vulnerable, unsure of where things were unravelling with regards my kidney as it was only weeks after this training that the transplant rejection began. One of the workshops was over two days, working with various inversions. It involved a lot of partner work so I had to trust a stranger, and they, in turn, had to trust me. I reached deeper levels of resilience through these experiences. It's not as simple as 'I'm fit and healthy and can do a handstand'. It's a willingness to surrender and literally turn yourself, and everything around you, on its head. One of the days I worked with a lovely South African lady.

We were guided into a challenging inversion, half hand-stand, half forearm balance, so one forearm was fully flat to the floor and the other the hand was completely flat, and that arm straight. All I wanted to say to my partner was, 'I can't do it. I haven't been well. My body has been through so much. I'm terrified. I'm going to sit this one out...'. Before I could start to speak, she just said calmly in her sweet Afrikans accent, "Come."

And I let go of the mind chatter, the stories, the fear pulling me into an ocean of despair, reached into that place of consistency, and trusted she would catch me if I fell. And I did it. Yoga offers us the capacity to move through the layers. To self-nurture. To be ok with what comes up. We learn to apply what is experienced on the mat to the day-to-day fabric of our lives. It gives to us the courage and confidence to explore our own deeply human experience so the 'I can't do it, I am absolutely terrified' can be transformed with support, in the blink of an eye, to 'Yes, yes you absolutely can.' That lovely woman will not know the true support she offered me that day. Never under estimate how you help others in what might seem a small act of kindness. We truly change the world in this way. Kindness heals.

Remember, too, that at its heart, yoga crosses so many landscapes of the human experience. It has become quite a showy, even luxury, lifestyle accessory in the West. It's a huge industry, with yoga studios, accessories, magazines, retreats and a mass presence on social media. Whilst it is a positive for its wisdom and teachings to be reaching greater numbers, we need to remember the ultimate premise is to provide a pathway to self-realisation. It is not an exercise class you attend once or twice a week in your fancy leggings, it is an opportunity to explore your true nature. This is not a whimsical, dreamy pursuit. This is bone-crushing honesty to strip yourself bare, bit by bit, each time you come to the mat. To look within. To check in. How am I today? What's making my mind race? Who am I underneath this cloak of stories? Who is the wearer of the cloak? Care enough for yourself to enquire about yourself, to yourself.

So the more we come to the mat and build a strong foundation of understanding, the more we can take this into our daily existence and routine. To help meet the challenges, the ups and downs, the mundane. Your yoga practise needs to serve you, otherwise why are you doing it?

An integral element of the yoga practise is the breath. We have this breath from the first gasp taken as a newborn, after being cocooned in the watery, warm solace of the womb. To the very last breath we exhale out in this body, as we expire. The exhale releases the soul from the limitations of the human body. The one constant in life is the breath. That is yours and yours alone. Get to know it well. Connect with it. Appreciate it.

Whilst breath is a part of our autonomic nervous system, meaning it happens voluntarily without us having to think about it, we also have the ability to influence it, to deepen it, to change it, to experience it. That makes it a very powerful tool to access our inner terrain.

I find it useful to use the analogy of thinking of the breath as a shower for the mind. A mental cleanser – alongside its physiological role of taking in oxygen and releasing carbon dioxide. We do not question the daily routine of washing our bodies so we feel clean and fresh, and don't smell. We must learn to apply that same daily diligence to our minds. The mind gets stinky and dirty too! Just it's not quite so obvious. It comes out in our behaviour, in our beliefs, in our choices. How clean is your behaviour? Are you wafting sweet aroma or are you letting off energetic stink bombs everywhere you go? How aware are you in the integrity of how you conduct yourself in your work, your relationships, or your encounters with strangers? This is self-enquiry. This is cleansing the mirror of the mind, the windows of your soul. This is being intimate with reality. It's not easy work, but it's worthwhile.

Yoga asana in a healthy body is wonderful. You build strength, lung capacity, feel more energised and discover new territory within your own anatomy. Health is not merely an absence of disease. If we believe as I do, that life is a mindset, we can decide we are indeed healthy and make it so – even though there may be things out of balance in the physical body. A healthy mind informs a healthy body and vice versa. Therefore, the more health and cleanliness we invite into the mind, the healthier we are able to become. As a whole in mind, body and spirit. And not in a puritanical way, but in a way that feels more hopeful and bright, alongside this significant re-awakening and unburdening.

This certainly rings true for me. For example, when I lost the remaining meaningful function in my transplant kidney and recovered from flu and chest sepsis, my physical body had gone through vast challenge. As I left hospital, ready to leave and to embrace the next chapter, I was still physically weak and adjusting to life with an abdominal catheter. There was physical pain in this area, my lungs were still sensitive, and I was short of breath after not much exertion. However, I adapted my yoga practise to accommodate this. I used meditation and regular visualisation of my body mending and healing. To begin with, I worked on just the upper body, opening up the shoulders. This felt so good after a week lying in a hospital bed.

So be where you're at with your practise. Adapt as needed. For example, if you have hypertension there are contraindications for some of the yoga poses, particularly inversions such as the headstand. This puts too much pressure on the baroreceptors in the neck, which are key feedback messaging ports for regulating blood pressure. I have in the past burst blood vessels in my eyes inverting in a hot studio – this was a lesson for me, as I should have known better than to perform a headstand in a small studio heated to almost 40 degrees Celsius! If you have a working fistula, be careful too of intense arm balances.

One of the absolute joys I've discovered in recent years is yin yoga. Yin yoga offers a deeply healing way to slow down. Where yang is a stronger and more dynamic aspect, yin is the antidote, offering the space to release deeply held tension and come away from muscular contraction in order to access our white connective tissue, the fascia. Yin is an invitation to become still and quiet. To just be. The poses are held for about five minutes or longer. They are passive, so as the seconds grow into minutes, the muscles are not in active contraction. They begin to soften, elongate and release, which perfuses into the surrounding fascia. It is also a rejuvenating practise for the joints. And keeping joints healthy is a key factor for wellbeing, given we have over two hundred in our body.

Of course, a significant challenge that comes with yin is in the allowing. If the body has gone through prolonged episodes of stress without considered recovery, it will battle this stillness as the mental agitation bubbles up. When the HPA (hypothalamus-pituitary-adrenal) axis is in overdrive, embracing stillness, may at first create unsettled feelings. Be patient. Give it time. Allow the old stories and patterns to start gently lifting away. Be with the discomfort, be with the tears – these are cleansers. As the rain relieves the skies from its heavy burdens, so too can the watery, salty tears provide relief from our own heaviness. Cry rivers of tears if that is what's needed for you. Again, I ask you to be intimate with reality.

The power of yin is something I wish to share and celebrate with as many as possible. This was such a welcome style of practise to discover and experience and it came - as these things often do - at a pivotal time in my spiritual development. It helped so much to look inwards and connect with the ability to feel.

When we start to dive more deeply into yin and yang, we discover much of it is subtle and contextual. For example, we could be breathing in a more yang, strong way, whilst holding a yin pose – so effectively we are always dancing in both the yin and the yang. What we are helping our bodies to do by holding these longer poses is to unravel and zoom into the deeper parts of us. As a pose is held, we move more towards a sense of surrender and release, and the deeper muscles and connective tissues have the opportunity to decompress. Now it's important, too, to understand yin yoga is not the same as restorative yoga – it is just a different way of moving into the experience of the body and mind. It can surface huge challenge in the mental realm as we move towards becoming still. This can be especially challenging for people who have disconnected from their bodies, or are living a punishing schedule and experiencing high levels of stress hormones, such as cortisol and adrenaline. Modern life has created such distraction in the external world. It's fast paced, demanding and rushed, with quick fixes, raised voices and aggravated communication. When we move into a place of stillness, the mind can still be extremely agitated, and that can show up in the physiological responses as well. It is so used to focussing outwards on external distractions, that the process of turning inwards can be tricky and challenging. This is why people often proclaim they have tried meditation and it didn't work for them. This is where patience, diligence and regularity come in to play. Know too these patterns can be changed. With discipline and an open heart, we can embrace what it really means to surrender, to soften, to release.

That is why yin yoga is so valuable. It becomes such a healing practise if we can move towards stillness and let the mind settle. Yin also helps us understand the energy body and the energy channels, as it draws upon Daoism, the foundation of traditional chinese medicine (TCM). This Chinese meridian system heavily influences the poses and how these specific yin poses help to open up and unblock these channels in the body, in a similar way to an acupressure session. In fact, I like to think of yin yoga as a self-acupressure session. You are using your own body to help open up and release blockages. Like the garden hose that has been lying unused for years, yin yoga helps you unblock the hose so water can flow through the temple of your body.

In TCM, organs in the body are in pairs, in a yin/yang relationship. For example: the kidney and bladder, heart and small intestine, lung and large intestine, liver and gallbladder. Meridians run throughout the body and are connected to the health of these organs. As we come to understand certain blocks or resistance in the body and where they might correlate to on the meridian map, we can harness better health for our organs. We can also look into the deeper aspects of what emotional and mental qualities correspond to different organs: an absorption issue in the small intestine could be reflective of an inability to absorb or assimilate certain situations. How are we soaking up life? A period of constipation, namely some aridity or a stuckness in the large intestine, could be an indication that you are struggling to let go of something. Literally and figuratively you need to just take a big dump! Rid yourself of an unnecessary burden. Lighten the load.

Yin is more connected with the energy of the moon, whereas yang is more connected to the sun's energy. This is actually a big premise of Hatha yoga too – Ha meaning sun and Tha meaning moon. But how do we interpret this? For me, this is, in part, about embracing our darkness. When the sun sets and the night comes to life, can we dance in the darkness of our experiences, or do we feel pulled into this darkness, terrified and rigid? To become whole, we must recognise we are yin and yang, of this darkness and light. If we don't begin to look at our shadow, it can take over. When we acknowledge our shadow - our darkness - we can ask, what can we learn from it? And then bring light, and disperse it. This is not easy work. But it is hugely important and transformational. We must do the inner work and spiritual excavation at an individual level, so we can heal the collective. Companies and institutions also have their shadow. Some are so entrenched in their shadow, they are damaging humanity. We must raise the vibration out of the turbulence and the destruction, to rise up as warriors of truth and exploration in order to overcome the underworld. Dare we love ourselves and our dear planet enough to do this? Yes. We must dare, whilst also keeping true to ourselves and to presence.

Yin can bring up old buried information, memories and experiences that we simply did not have the capacity or tools to deal with at the time. But for a trauma to be healed, it first needs to be witnessed, so it can then be brought into our conscious awareness to be released. In yin yoga, a major premise is to track physical sensation. This does mean discomfort at times. But this needs to be at a level you can manage and that keeps the breath flowing. Life is, at times, uncomfortable. How can we make ourselves more comfortable with our own discomfort? One way is to bring awareness to what discomfort there is. And yin allows this exploration.

Come out of the fear, move into here.

Yoga offers such a bedrock upon which to build a strong and stable foundation. A strong, healthy body means a greater likelihood of a strong, healthy mind. Greater flexibility in the body equals greater flexibility in the mind. It's all connected.

We must be attentive to our mental rigidity. A common statement I hear from people being reluctant to take up a yoga practise is, 'I'm not flexible enough.' That's quite a statement to make about yourself. Yoga is not a pursuit of bendiness and gymnastic tricks. It is a journey inwards. Sometimes the practise is coming to the mat and just lying in savasana. Sometimes it is weeping. Being with the tears. Sometimes it is jubilant. It changes. We need to continually ask ourselves, what is really happening when we are practising yoga? The more expansive your knowledge of your own physiology and anatomy, the more you will come to understand how powerful it is, as a catalysing transformation on all levels. I am frequently surprised at people's own limited knowledge of their bodies: for example, one educated young woman in one of my group classes did not know where her adrenal glands were. We have a plethora of topics in life to study, yet many are not familiar with their own structure and form. You begin a very beautiful dance with a meaningful spiritual form of activity such as yoga, ecstatic dance, Qi gong or walking in nature. Yoga is not the only tool – it just happens to be one I love!

I'd also like to talk about Shamanic wisdom. For some, the very mention of the word 'shaman' invokes fear and suspicion, and a bit of confusion. Even Parley has a view that shamans were manipulative and hungry for power. I have no idea how this emerged, as this is very much not my experience of it, and I'd like to share its innate beauty and wisdom with you. I'm sure in the past there have been people who have manipulated their position in the community, but sadly this happens across cultures and continues to this day in various guises.

In many cultures, the shaman has been the pivotal healer within the community. They would go beyond the tangible and physical worlds, into the unseen, and help people uncover the root of their maladies. In recent years, I have dived deeper into the Peruvian lineage of shamanic wisdom in particular. My month-long yoga training in Peru had a significant Shamanic arm to it, so I explored this particular lineage more than others. In fact, here this is known more as the Curendero rather than the shaman, but we can consider the term as interchangeable for now.

I don't recall specifically when I came to be interested in this. In Zambia, I used to absolutely love and be fascinated by chameleons. How fortunate were the rare occasions I would find one in our garden, always camouflaged in a tree. I remember one time I caressed the chameleon gently from its branch and arranged a big box with some banana leaves for it. I was thrilled to be so close to this creature. I took it into the house to be greeted by a giant screech from our housekeeper, Grace. I was quite aghast and Marley came quickly to the kitchen, to investigate the commotion. Grace did not at all like the chameleon and I think the local folklore holds far more suspicions of these animals. So I had to put it back into the garden (rightly so in hindsight, as it would not have been fair to have kept him). Years later, I discovered one of my power animals was a chameleon – so my connection with them made much more sense. Discovering aspects of an animal, and how their characteristics might call and help you, is magical. All is an expression of life.

Shamanic wisdom, like so many of the ancient teachings, inspires us to connect more deeply with the laws of nature. So, what does that really mean in our modern setting? Consider your own life for a moment and how much time you spend in natural daylight, versus how much you spend in front of a screen, be it television, smart phone, laptop or computer. We evolved in the wisdom of the elements, not hypnotised in front of a screen. Now, I'm not saying that all this technology is bad. Through self-discovery, we know not to necessarily judge things as good or bad, just to view them as they are. For me, I like to feel free and not at the mercy of technology. Yes, it's super that I can quickly look up a train time and figure out a journey route with little effort. But I have no desire to become absorbed in these things for long periods, or be consumed by them. I want to be in my body and experience the richness of each moment as much as possible. For me, cruising persistently on screens does not enhance my life –I see it do the very opposite for a lot of people. It's a fast track route to isolation. What I find utterly extraordinary is that we are exposed to more now in one single day than our ancestors were in a whole lifetime. That is just mind blowing. And it's little wonder that our kids are more stressed than ever. It's a tricky time to be growing up. We need to remember that the magnificent simplicity of coming back to nature can ease so much. To sit by an oak tree, to swim in the ocean, to raise our arms to the sun, to feel the grassy meadow beneath our feet. Let's not lose this rich simplicity.

Shamanism and yoga share much in common in terms of the deeper messaging. One of the ideas I love to connect with is shape shifting. I like to think of shape shifting as bringing us to the present as much as possible. We morph into our environment and respond swiftly to changes, without drama. In the asana practise of yoga, the practise of the poses, we shape shift physically to experience ourselves in all kinds of positions. To marinate in revelation through the language of sensation.

When we choose to explore nature and ourselves more deeply, magic begins to reveal itself. Magic, in essence, is bringing thought to form –

to create our own reality through the power of our higher mind and our five senses. Dare we believe in the brilliance of what it is to be alive? There is so much to explore.

The power of circle is very much respected in the Peruvian Curendero tradition. At the outset of our training in the Sacred Valley of Peru, we formed a circle and set a group intention for our time together: pay attention to what we pay attention to. Spending a month being reminded and aware of that was incredible for opening up to how much our mental patterns and fluctuations impact our own wellbeing.

I had not managed to ease off my daily dose of morning coffee ahead of the training and knew it was unlikely coffee would be on offer. So, knowing my body well, I braced myself for the withdrawal– typically I get a dreadful headache and feel pretty rotten for a day or so. This came the following day and I felt awful. Nauseous alongside the bad headache. As we had created the circle and agreed to bring our best selves to this place each day, I felt I had to go to morning practise. All I could do was sit, whilst everyone else moved through their asana practise. Even attempting a child's pose made me feel sick. So, I sat, wrapped in a blanket, for two hours. Staying in my breath when I felt waves of nausea. It was a humbling experience to recognise that this sitting was my practise for that day. Sitting and marinating in my unwellness, without becoming overwhelmed by it, while showing up energetically for the group. I'm sure there was more at play than just the coffee withdrawal. I was embarking on a significant journey, physically and emotionally. We were all adjusting too to the high altitude and breath was quite short and laboured due to this.

Our training was run from the heart by the main teacher, CJ Ananda. We were showered with gifts through the month – rattles, pens, trips to the mountains, cacoa and mala beads. Such generosity. We were held truly in a space of love and honest exploration.

Quite early into the training in one of our classes, CJ asked us to consider: "What are you doing here? What the fuck are you doing here?"

We laughed at the expletive, but it was useful to reflect on that. To consider what work we had come to do for ourselves. As I explained in Chapter 3, in the lead up to going to Peru and increasingly whilst there, I kept hearing the word 'dialysis' in my mind. It started coming through very clearly and often. This was at the time I had about sixteen per cent function remaining in the kidney and there was the big, looming question of 'what next?'. These whisperings were an invitation for me to keep facing my fears.

One morning after our yoga practise and breakfast, CJ announced, "We are doing a sweat lodge today!" This was exciting, but I also noticed a sense of immediate unease rise up in my belly, never having done one before. I felt fearful. Traditional sweat lodges are not for the faint hearted – and arguably not for those with compromised renal function, as I was to discover. However, I always wish to explore experiences and check myself when I feel fear is driving the choice. Yes, I felt a bit scared, but I still wanted to step into the adventure. Also, sweating releases plenty of toxins –some even call the skin the third kidney, as we can rid our self of a lot though the skin. This was a comforting thought. A Mexican and his companion facilitated the sweat lodge ritual.

As with all of the important processes we experienced in Peru, this ritual was highly revered. The lodge had been prepared during the day for a night-time ritual, after the sun had set. The intensity of the daytime heat would have been far too much. The lodge was simple, yet effective, in its construction. Made with wood, it was similar to a wigwam, but not as high. Over the wood foundation, heavy alpaca wool blankets were draped so not even a smidgen of air could get in or out. It is heated by hot rocks that have been burning for hours ahead of the ceremony and start as a fairly small pile that get added to after the end of each hour, and the group sings to the rocks to welcome them. We were advised to dress lightly and to feel free to partake naked in the ritual, which some chose to do. I had on only a pair of pants and a sarong wrapped around me. We called in the cardinal directions and spirit guides from a place of open heartedness, setting the intention that it would be a safe space. About 20 of us went inside, one-by-one. We all sat in a circle towards the edges and it was cosy to say the least. The blanket doorway was brought down to seal the lodge. It was dark. We had our rattles and began to shake them to create a rhythm, while the Mexican chanted. As the chanting subsided we were encouraged to share, one-by-one, what we wanted to let go of – and, indeed, anything else we felt compelled to say out loud. I can't recall exactly what I said during this first round, but I was already feeling emotional and things were shifting within my energy. It was almost euphoric at points. One of the young men in our group was visibly struggling with the heat and we were all sending him good vibes. There was a bit of pressure to feel like you can beat the heat – but it is hugely overwhelming and so I completely understood why he had to leave. This was just the first hour – the ceremony was set to last for four hours. At the end of each hour, the blanket was pulled open and the fresh air felt so good, and was such a relief. We could go outside for a short period, if we needed to, and drink water, which was not allowed inside the sweat lodge, aside from it being poured onto the hot rocks in the centre of the circle. So, basically, the heat intensifies more and more. By the middle of the first round I could not care less about modesty and had removed the sarong and sat, a hot sweaty mess, in just my pair of pants. Sweat was pouring off all of us.

The second round started after our very brief respite and we began the chanting, shaking the rattles and sharing again. I could feel the initial euphoria moving into massive over-heating and felt like I would pass out. I sat it out for a while, seeing if I could breathe through it. My face felt like it was on fire. After what seemed like a number of minutes, I had to speak out and said to the person sitting next to me, "I think I'm going to pass out."

He said to lie down and place my face at the bottom as some small pockets of air might come through. I was digging deep here, but at the same time fading fast. I tried the lying down but remained overwhelmed and I had to get out. I managed two rounds and that was enough for me. I left a wreck, literally crawling and crying out of there on all fours, grateful for the life in my body. I commend the remaining people who lasted the whole four rounds, and could hear the yelps of delight from the communal area as they threw themselves into the cold river as the ceremony completed. There were a few others who had to leave halfway too, and I was glad to have honoured the messaging from my body. It is said you die to yourself in a sweat lodge. There is nowhere to hide. You are there, and exposed and sweating. It's no place for niceties and 'I'm fine'. It's raw, visceral and hot, and in some ways utterly glorious – even with the waves of discomfort it brings. I certainly had a mini death and if I'd pushed it much further, I might actually have done my health a great disservice. I graciously bowed out of the next sweat lodge a few days later.

This extraordinary month in the Andes, immersed in shamanic, Ayurvedic and yogic wisdom alongside likeminded people, was a profound experience. We'd also learned about the medicine wheel of the Andes, and it was now in my psyche, so when I returned home I discovered a wondrous online course facilitated by the amazing Shift Network, offered by an incredible Peruvian Curendero, Don Oscar Miro Quesada. I embarked on the first training, entitled *The Universal Path of the Shaman*. Don Oscar had received messages from the Elders that now was the time to be sharing this precious ancient wisdom, to help heal Earth and its people, and to remind us of our intricate relationships with nature. Such elegance and symbolism. I loved this course so much that I immediately signed up for the next one, *Magic, Mysticism and Medicine*. Although these were online courses, they were so personal and broadcast from Don Oscar's own home and mesa. Through these courses we built our own mesa, or altar, which is, in essence, a deep reflection of the cosmos and the forces contained within in. We were guided through magnificent rituals and it was very much a combination of wisdom information, together with the experience. For example, doing the rituals and making poultices and burying our wounds. He helped me feel, explore and understand this magic for myself and I started to weave some of this medicine into my own teachings.

I ran workshops with a shamanic angle, such as *Flight of the Eagle,* to help connect more with spirit, and *Journey with the Serpent,* to look more at our physical form.

I have learned, through my interest in shamanic wisdom, to connect more with nature and with dreamtime. How healing it can be to sit beneath an old oak tree and drink in its rooted wisdom. In shamanism, there is a great interest in nature and observing the laws of nature, and the Hermetic principles. This includes connecting more with the wisdom of animals and helping you discover which power animals walk with you in your lifetime. You can consider a power animal as an animal that you really resonate with, or whose particular qualities you need to draw upon for a certain situation. Indeed, you might have one particular animal that you resonate with, or that visits you in dreams with messages. Over the past three years or so, since connecting more with shamanic wisdom, I have experienced some notable and memorable dreams. One saw me sitting in a garden shed and noticing a large black hair coming out of my chin. I pulled at it and it came out completely, after which I cast it to the floor where it transformed into a plume of smoke rising from the ground, before morphing into a shiny black snake that unfurled its way out into a very ornate looking garden. I subsequently learned that snakes represent our physical body in one of the medicine wheels of the Andes. They also represent wisdom and exploring the darker aspects of ourselves – if you consider that, typically, snakes like to curl up in dark places. Be open to decoding the messages that come to you in dreamtime. Interestingly, the point on my chin where I pulled the hair from corresponds to the kidneys, and snakes represent the healing of the physical body.

Another dream I had was of a big mother bear. She was very distressed and crying, while wandering quite restlessly outside what looked like a big lodge on a mountainside. Humans were coming out of this lodge, running and screaming in terror because of the bear. I looked it up in my animal medicine book the next day, to find that the bear represents introspection, and it also made reference to the Dream Lodge in the description of bear. This lovely book was a gift from a past client and it holds details and stories of many animals. Each animal has one trait that is strongly associated with it, represented in one word, so, for the bear, it was Introspection; I interpreted this as the dream telling me about the Dream Lodge. The energy of bear wishes to hold us in introspection and reflection, and to celebrate our dream state. It did feel at some level that in my dream, bear was heartbroken for humanity and how we have come to fear our own capacity to dream. I absolutely love what the dream state can offer us in terms of understanding. Sometimes the messages are visionary and deep, sometimes a playing out of the sub-conscious. And, of course, it's up to you how you interpret and decode them. There are no fixed rules here, just intuition and exploration.

Another dream I had was of a dolphin. I had come into what I think was a bedroom and, looking out of a big floor-to-ceiling window, could see a large dolphin floating in the air outside. The dolphin actually seemed completely content, but I was concerned as it was out of its usual seawater home. I recall Parley then being in my dream and helping me to get the dolphin inside, where we started to splash water on it. This panned to an image of us putting the dolphin in a bath, where it transformed into a man. The next day I watched the Luc Besson film Lucy, which contained a reference to dolphins together with a much deeper, spiritual message of how much wisdom and connection humans are capable of, and how we use only ten per cent of our brain capacity. In shamanic wisdom, the dolphin represents Manna, as per that same lovely book I mentioned, which means the life force or breath. Did I need to connect more with my own breath and life force? Most likely, yes. What a valuable message to come through.

As an aside, dolphins use twenty per cent of their brain capacity; whilst that is still a long way off 100 per cent, surely we humans can increase our capacity? The dream also speaks to the shape shifting of forms, from dolphin to man. Shape shifting is a natural part of our creativity. We see this in people like actors and dancers, who effortlessly change form. But we all have access to it. When we hone it as a skill, we can adapt swiftly to any situation. To me shape shifting is presence.

Another dream actually made me feel scared. You know those dreams when you wake and have wobbly leg sensation? I dreamed very clearly that two big lions had appeared in my home. They had a strong presence and I was terrified. I ran upstairs to escape, but had the feeling one was pursuing me. I creaked a door open to see one of them was sleeping in a bedroom. I went to barricade myself into the next bedroom, but found that the window was broken and I had a feeling they would get in that way. The dream ended there, and I woke up very unsettled. As I chose fear in the dream instead of pausing to look or talk to the lions, I feel I missed out from receiving more of their wisdom. Upon reflection, whilst their presence was strong and commanding, I don't believe they really would have hurt me. I then started to receive a message, 'Follow the lions.' And I began to notice lion imagery and statues all over the place in my day-to-day life. I don't believe it was a coincidence that I then came across Celia Fenn online, who was running four webinars to bring in the energy of the Lionsgate portal, which I signed up for. This transpired to be extraordinary and helped me understand more how, as humanity, we are moving through a very potent time, and we can connect more with our experiences. Celia Fenn lives in South Africa, so it was also helpful to reconnect with lion country. It then, of course, made complete sense why the lions had visited me in dream-space. To encourage me. To IN COURAGE me to tap into their lion hearts and strength.

I believe in the deep yearning for goodness that humanity has. That is our natural state. All the layers and insanity smother this natural state. Our stories, our deceptions and untruths keep us out of the bliss within. Dare we reveal who we truly are? YES! What is the value of remaining hidden? Shine your light. I commit to shining my light, so together we all switch on each other's lights.

For me, yoga is that powerful tool which helps us remember our natural state. But there are so many tools. Bodywork, Qi Gong, music, dance, hiking. Find yours. Do things you love and are naturally drawn towards. So on those days you feel, 'Urrgh, not today', you can feel into the experienced benefits and motivate yourself for tomorrow, or the day after that.

Life is a puzzle. Yoga helps us put the puzzle together, so all the edges meet.

Top tips for yoga

- Start somewhere. Find a local class, or if you attend a gym, find out if it runs one. Experiment with different classes and teachers until you find the one, or ones, that work for you. If funds are an issue, YouTube is a great resource for free classes. Books can also be super ways to enrich your understanding. Or, talk to friends or people you know who are practising yoga and see what they say. Yogaglo is also a good online resource and offers a free introductory trial, as do most yoga studios. So, enjoy exploring! You are also most welcome to check out my own YouTube channel: Wholly Aligned.

- Remain open. If your first class is not a good experience, don't be put off. Keep seeking out what does work for you. Every teacher brings their own style and personality, so there will be someone to suit you.

- Ask your GP about social prescribing and what is available to you through that, as yoga is at the precipice of becoming fully integrated into the NHS.

- Yin and Yang in life is important. As you explore your practise, be aware to explore both of those aspects. Strength and softness. Masculine and feminine. Sun and moon.

- Let the breath always be your constant companion. Building a relationship with your own breath means you tune into it every day. Presence with the breath anchors us into our bodies and out of chaotic thought patterns. It is a process and a practise.

- Do ask questions of your teachers if you are unsure if the level of class is suitable for you, or if you are working with an injury or health issue. It will help begin a dialogue of enquiry to enhance your own journey into self discovery. Teachers, for the most part, are extremely knowledgeable and will offer modifications and guidance personal to you. Make the most of that! The teacher wants to serve you in the best way.

- Release the temptation to compare. Each person is on their own journey. One road to misery is to compare yourself to others. It's fine to be aware of how other people are practising, but with an objective eye rather than one of comparison, or wishful thinking.

- Know that stuff comes up on the mat. Some days your practise will be effortless and enjoyable. Some days you might leave feeling heavy and the body fatigued. That is the mirror of life. The emphasis becomes more and more on observing your experience. What is really going on here? Why do I feel this way? How did I get to this space? What part of my body am I experiencing? I was at a wonderful yin class with a beautiful teacher, Emma Peel, and a lady began to cry. Quite open and audible sobs. We were working deep into the hips. From my perspective, this was such a positive experience to be part of, and for others in the class to see and witness - it's ok to feel your feelings. The teacher went to be next to the crying lady who simply said "It's just so sad." She cried for some time and I have no doubt this was a profound shifting of something for her. This is enormously brave. Gift yourself that permission to be with what comes up.

- Practise on an empty stomach to avoid compromising the digestive process, or feeling uncomfortable with a full belly. These days I leave at least three hours before practise, unless it is something very light.

- Make the most of savasana (final relaxation) at the end of the class. This is such a key part of the practise; in time, it will help you feel more and more settled within yourself, and teach you how to pour yourself more into stillness. Savasana translates to corpse pose, and is a reminder of the cyclical nature of life and death. We live, we die. Dare we embrace our death to live fully, to be wholly alive?

- Keep exploring. Even if you have been practising for years, remain curious and keep diving into your experience with fresh eyes.

- Experience several teachers. There are so many wonderful teachers across the globe. And they all have their own unique gift and perspective to share with you. So even if you have a favourite, be open to attending workshops and courses with others.

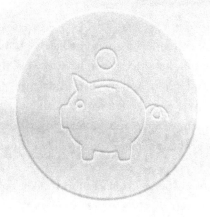

CHAPTER SIX

Your Wellbeing Fund

This idea of a wellbeing fund came to me after working for a long time in private banking. For the more logical and left brained among you, I hope this helps to connect more with the variables that make up your experience of life. And for the more right brained creatives, that it provides a framework which is helpful and practical.

How we invest our money, or 'wealth management' as it is often referred to in a private banking sense, is important. Well, actually… how we are investing in our health is also of the utmost importance. How about our 'health management'? What credits have you been building up to create a meaningful wellbeing fund? If the investment has been little, or even zero, when a crisis comes along there are no meaningful reserves to draw upon. And so we develop a negative value in our wellbeing fund, which is much harder to recover from — especially if we have the expectation that the solutions lie solely in pharmaceuticals. A bit like starting your day with a strong cup of coffee – you are immediately putting your body in a hydration deficit. From that place it will have to work much harder and already be in stimulation mode. If we instead start the day with hot water and lemon, and then have the coffee with a small bit of food so it doesn't spike an adrenaline surge, this is much better. It's all about understanding how your patterns grow or deplete your wellbeing fund.

Money is one solution when it comes to investment. So how we spend our money is important, as is how much we earn. What proportion of our income do we spend on good, wholesome food, on a massage, or on enjoying a glass of wine with friends? Chasing money as the solution to our problems is a big trap that many fall into. Part of becoming wholly aligned is to really ask what our relationship with money is, and how that links in with our own value system. There is nothing wrong with earning a lot of money. What you are doing with it is the more relevant – and indeed, revealing – component.

I remember talking with my sister about credibility at work. She made a very valid point about challenging work situations and dealing with perceived incompetent or thoughtless behaviour. In the corporate environment, I tended to be a 'say it like it is' person. I have an honest and direct approach, so my words would reflect my mood; at times because I felt the burden of attempting to be the self-imposed, moral compass in situations. I would get very frustrated, annoyed and irritated. Frankly flabbergasted. Of course these situations were great learning curves, although at the time I did not yet know it!

My sister was saying that you can get away with certain bad behaviour; many people get annoyed with their boss, and will be a bit short with them if they don't agree with what they are saying. But if you have overall built up a strong and credible relationship, those moments of irritation, annoyance or abruptness are accepted and will rarely impact the overall relationship. Because the credibility is there. If no credibility was there, such an instance would potentially jeopardise your reputation and you might be seen as volatile. It's all about the context. Further reflection on these scenarios has helped me understand much more that everyone needs to feel safe and appreciated in their work role. This is a big reason why I had to listen to the call of my soul and leave the corporate world, as it was not where I could thrive. Now, this absolutely does not mean that others cannot thrive in that same environment. Some can be the shining lights in such a place and it suits them. You need to decide. But first you need some honesty and reflection. Allow this chapter to be that for you. Dive into the interactive part and self-enquire.

When we apply this same thought process of credibility to your health, we can discover what our own relationship is with health credibility. Consider: how have you been raised or influenced to build credit and invest in your own health? If you had poor self-care modelled to you by your immediate family, give yourself the chance to acknowledge that, and choose another path that is truer to yourself and where you are now.

Consider how much money directly influences culture. It is just one cog in the wheel. 'Culture is how we do things round here' is a phrase coined by the McKinsey organisation, which it sums up well. A culture of respect, self-worth, support, encouragement – these are deeply positive and nurturing human behaviours that are part of the fabric of a place, be it within a company, a village, a city or a person. People need to feel valued, heard and supported in their environment, be it in the workplace, their family or intimate relationships. There is a movement in leadership for leaders and managers to have more of an outlook of service to their staff. To ask more of their staff, "How can I serve you?" Instead of this outdated model of command and control. So might you ask – how can I serve myself, rather than expecting everything to run in an orderly way, dictated from an established hierarchy of power?

We could also apply the thought process of the wellbeing fund to wider organisations. So yes, it's absolutely valid in an individual sense, but how about applying the philosophy to the NHS, for example? If we unpick the statistics of the NHS in terms of job satisfaction, staff sickness and suicide risk, we might find its wellbeing fund is severely depleted. Finding meaningful ways to replenish this would serve the public greatly, as well as employees, from the administration staff to the chief surgeons. Remember, our current systems are all a part of our collective consciousness. We all contributed to their making in some way.

Here's what a balanced wellbeing fund might look like:

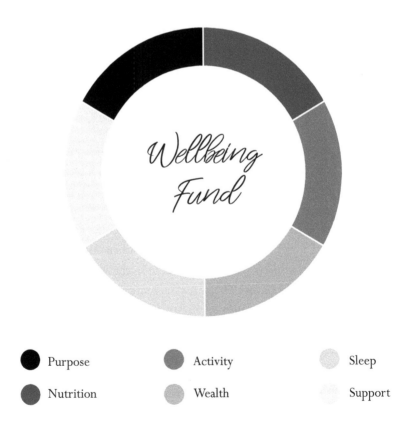

| ● Purpose | ● Activity | ● Sleep |
| ● Nutrition | ● Wealth | ● Support |

Exploration of the categories

Remember, this is a dynamic and interlinked concept. And that all facets of the fund will feed each other: for example, our self-worth is linked to our beliefs around money. How we nourish ourselves physically through food will influence our capacity to be active and enjoy movement. Everything influences everything, all of the time. We can also consider self worth as very much linked to wellbeing. A depleted wellbeing fund is likely to come with lower self esteem.

The wellbeing fund will vary depending on your life stage and individual circumstances. It is not a linear situation, as life is always changing. It is dynamic and fluid, not rigid.

DHARMA/PURPOSE

The concept of Dharma is that your life is purposeful as an expression of conscious awareness. This doesn't mean the mind can 'figure' out your purpose. When we surrender the mind, and step into presence, we are more likely to see and feel clearly the signs pointing to our purpose. We will access the innate knowledge that we are doing what we have come to this earth to do. We see this in people around us, who are naturally doing what they love because they have not questioned, or fretted, about it. They have simply known, from a place within, that this is what they are here to do. I'm sure we can all bring to mind someone we know who is doing what they love.

For me, it is much clearer now that I have walked through the alchemical fire of this health journey, come out all the stronger, and be able to inspire and share my story with others, for the greater good. And this purpose absolutely feels right in my bones. Are there other ways I live a purposeful life? Of course! The beauty starts to be revealed when we attend more to what we love and enjoy from a place of openness, rather than blame or judgement.

One of the most powerful moments for me in recent years was vocalising to a group of women, 'I am ready to go big.' We were in the open-plan kitchen area of a friend's home in South London, and she was embarking on a new endeavour, facilitating a womens' group. I helped gather some people for her, including myself! After setting the scene, the facilitator asked us to go as deep as possible, and we went around the table sharing where we were at in life, and whatever else we wished. People were sharing, but to some extent, keeping an emotional lid on themselves. How often we present just the surface of what we truly feel. That day, I had received the green light to be listed for a second kidney transplant and was in an already heightened emotional state. As my turn ebbed closer my heart rate was increasing, as I knew that from a visceral place, I had to dig deep and speak from the heart. I had to not hold back and brush over where I was and how I was feeling, as might have been my pattern in the past. My turn came and my voice already was shaking. The words formed from deep inside: "I am ready to go big…but fear holds me back."

And the tears came. The emotion of it all was too much, so they simply had to spill. It was a brief wobble and I re-vocalised my desire to go big, and received tremendous support and encouragement from the facilitator. This then allowed the lovely woman next to me to also step into her vulnerability; she also began to cry when she shared her story. She was feeling overwhelmed in her job as a solicitor, along with the angst of wishing to have a child with her husband, but it just wasn't happening. We serve others by sharing truthfully. We open the door to give permission to self-express. After that evening, more wonderful opportunities started to flow. I was featured in Yoga Magazine and the Journal of Kidney Care, and contributed to a psychology self-help manual, written by a young Italian PhD Psychology student in the neuroscience department at Guys Hospital. This has led to more collaboration between us, and we are going to embark on sharing ideas to help medical staff and their wellbeing, through combining psychology and yoga. When you crack your heart open, the doors of possibilities open wide. This then allows you, more and more, to step into your purposeful life. To me, that is what being in your dharma is. Open and willing.

Living a purposeful life could be as simple as bringing awareness to the left and right side of your brain, and how coordinated and harmonised they are. This takes things right back to evolutionary basics. We evolved with a negative bias within the left hemisphere of the brain, in order to protect our gene pool by sensing fear and running from life threatening situations. Of course, this 'survival instinct' has been massively over-stimulated by agitating aspects of modern life, that leave us rushing and often checked out of our bodies. This means the negative bias is leading to destruction, rather than evolutionary protection.

A very helpful way to connect with a sense of purpose in life, is to set the tone for each day. This is where skillfulness in action really comes into play. And playfulness is an important component. We are creative beings and life is intended to be playful and exploratory, at least sometimes. Setting the tone upon rising each day could be as simple as gazing momentarily upon something beautiful. This is actually a part of dinacharya in Ayurveda and it makes complete sense to me. I am fortunate to live right by a small forest, so as I draw back my curtains, I drink in the green trees that bow to me each morning. Compare this to rushing out of bed in a panic and full of anxious thoughts. That is setting the tone for the day. Change your habits, change your life.

We can then apply this from a daily ritual to different chapters in our life, so we can set the tone for a whole chapter. For example, in your first pregnancy, set the tone to take each day as it comes and trust the generational wisdom contained within your cells. I also find it incredibly helpful to set the tone through intentions at the beginning of the year: I meditate upon three words that resonate for me on New Years' Eve. I often include deep reflection on the previous year and the myriad of things that I am grateful for. It's so powerful. We change the fabric of our very beings in this simple way. Human life is complicated because we have made it so. What we truly require to thrive is wonderfully simple.

The gift of serving others can be such deep and profound medicine. Placing a genuine and heartfelt focus on an individual, a cause, a group, or service to others is deeply nurturing and deeply healing, both for the receiving party and for the giver. I certainly experienced this when going through losing the function of Kenny. Going to teach yoga classes during that time was so beneficial, as it took me out of the worry and fret and into service and a bigger picture. There were others who needed to receive. I had that strong sense of purpose which was, frankly, a life-saver.

Reflection on purpose and living a purposeful life

When I am true to myself, I am strong beyond measure. Say this out loud. How does it feel, and where do you feel it?

What does it mean to you to live a purposeful life?

What are you ready for? How can you be more ready? It's ok to do things in steps and stages.

ACTIVITY & MOVEMENT

Moving our bodies helps to release stagnation and to feel what the body is saying to you. The body is always communicating to you, so moving it well opens up your own channels of somatic exploration. As long as we take shape and form in a human body, this will be so. The more you can attune and feel, the more you can respond consciously to these communication signals. Movement can be what is enjoyable to you. There are so many options out there. For me, I love the freedom of freestyle dance to inspirational music, especially if it has powerful drum beats. Of course, yoga is also a huge part of my activity and movement routine. I also love to go on big country walks. This stems, I believe, from Parley being a keen walker. To this day, well into his seventies, he takes to the fields and walks for miles every week. Not only is this a lovely way to move the body without unnecessary stress on the joints, it also brings us out into nature and into the arms of the elements. We can feel the breeze, the solidity of earth beneath our feet, and the sun on our crowns.

I include bodywork in the activity and movement section of the wellbeing fund. I am a huge fan of regular bodywork and go for weekly massages and monthly reflexology sessions, as well as regular swaps with a lovely osteopath. I did not have very positive experiences in mainstream medicine in relation to activity and movement. The only very basic interaction I had with a physiotherapist was a two minute conversation, when I had my working transplant annual review around exercise. I have always been active, so this encounter was not added value to me. There needs to be hands on sessions available. In 2016, after I had the catheter fitted, I had no physio advice from the hospital when, arguably, this was when I needed it most. The nurses just mentioned to lift no more than 10kgs and avoid abdominal exercise – extremely limited advice. Because I already had established abdominal strength, it would serve my posture, breathing and overall wellbeing much better to maintain that. I have had no issues with deep abdominal activity, including learning the static trapeze and practising inversions, such as headstands and handstands, whilst having the catheter and dialysis fluid inside my peritoneal cavity. This also applies to the advice to lift no more than 10kgs. At the time I weighed about 46kgs, so that's over one fifth of my body weight. To a 6ft tall man who weighs 90kgs, 10 kgs is not much. So, my view is that it needs to be relative. I gave this feedback to a physiotherapist who interviewed me as part of a research project, exploring how culture influences exercise. I reference this as an example, because when people have been ill or had surgery, there can be a fear of moving. The body needs to move and lubricate itself – so keep tuning into your inner physician as to what feels right. This isn't about disregarding other professional advice, but be discerning about who has given it to you and if they have truly understood the context.

As I continued to work on strength, I joined a static trapeze class. The teacher was aware of the catheter as it was important, so we just avoided front balances. It was the most physically challenging thing I have ever done and much of it engages the core deeply. This has not been an issue for the catheter at all. This, however, is based on how I feel and the strength I already had cultivated in my body, so it might not make sense for everyone to be jumping onto a trapeze!

Moving our bodies is so key to wellness. It's super for releasing stress and deepening the breath which helps tone the whole system and we breathe more effectively. Muscle mass is also important to health as it is more metabolically active and keeps us strong and less likely to injury through falls. This is especially true as we grow older.

Under this activity section, I would include your own personal interests. Music and dance, cookery, sports, and even languages, are all part of that. For me, my soul is nourished when I sing and dance. I love the freedom of moving my body, and know in my very being how both have been my own saviours. I can dance my way out of pain, I can move with desire, I can feel the anger and explode it into strong movement. I am reminded of the strength of my body this way.

Of course, sexual intimacy can also be captured under activity. Sacred sexual union is our birthright, yet many never experience it – or realise they can. To truly embody oneself and another in a naked embrace, where each is bearing witness and engaging, not only from a place of sexual desire, but from a place of heart and connection. It is interesting that many marriages are now without this intimacy. The initial burning flames of passion fall away. It requires ongoing and honest communication. I did experience this with my long-term partner when I was in my twenties.

It was probably one of the reasons I felt so bereft when that relationship ended, as we had connected very deeply at that level and it happened very naturally. It was also probably a big reason for remaining in the relationship, because that part was so good. That is certainly an ongoing lesson for me. With subsequent partners I have not been in love with, I have not had that deeper connection.

Reflection on Activity/Movement

What movement and activity do you enjoy?

How can you incorporate what you enjoy into your life?

Based on your culture and upbringing, what are your beliefs around what good activity levels are?

SLEEP

This is such a pillar of health that it simply must feature in the wellbeing fund. And actually, when this piece of your pie is out of balance, it's highly likely the rest will be – and, certainly, your wellbeing fund will start to be extremely depleted. The increasing fast pace and demands we place on ourselves has massively undermined how pivotal a good night's sleep is. We must sleep enough. Poor sleep will show up in all sorts of ways. It will generally impact mood and make you more likely to reach for fast carbs for a quick hit of glucose. This becomes a cycle of persistent blood sugar spikes, which not only stresses the pancreas but also the adrenals. Big energy crashes are also more likely as the body attempts to stabilise. We then start relying too much on caffeine to prop us up – this is all a recipe for burnout. Of course, your body is always communicating to you, so burnout means many previous signals have been ignored, or not sufficiently understood. This isn't about blaming anyone, including yourself: it's about opening your mind to better ways of life. I do believe many mental health issues would be resolved from addressing sleep. Having a bedtime routine is helpful, in that it indicates to your nervous system that rest is coming. So avoid violent TV programs, including the news, before going to bed. Have clear boundaries with electronics and resist bringing any electronic devices into the haven of your bedroom. Such devices are too mentally stimulating and are the opposite signal to restfulness.

Reflection on sleep

What is your current quality of sleep? Consider how many hours per night you get and any disturbances.

Do you have a bedtime routine? What are you ready to change around this if you do not?

What disturbs your sleep and is that a modifiable factor? For example, alcohol.

Are the practical aspects of your sleep conducive? For example, cotton bedding, cool temperature, calm and clear bedroom environment. Creating a space that reflects rest and peace is helpful. You then wake up to pleasant surroundings, rather than mess.

NUTRITION CHOICES

Another key pillar of your wellbeing fund. I emphasise again there is no one size fits all, and what works for one chapter of your life might need a complete re-shift in another. I love the motto 'Eat food, not too much, mostly plants', from author Michael Pollan. It sums nutrition up beautifully.

Everything that passes our lips, aside from water, is considered a digestive event. Nutritional medicine goes far beyond just the food we eat – we need to explore the entire food chain. We know commercial farming has had a depletive effect on the soil and, sadly, much terrain has been polluted by persistent organic phosphates. We cannot continue to remain disembodied from how our food comes to be on our plates and expect our bodies - or, indeed, our planet - to heal. The more we heal our bodies, the more we heal our collective. Nutrition also encompasses a representation of how much we value ourselves. It is also a deep expression of how we interact with our own environment. Remember, there is no one protocol that works for everyone. Tune into what foods energise you and make your body and mind feel well.

Please refer to the Top Tips section at the end of the chapter on Nutrition for the reflective component on this. Go through those suggestions and notice how they make you feel.

WEALTH/FINANCIAL SECURITY/ACCESS TO FLOW OF CURRENCY

Our basic needs require satisfying in order to feel safe and to then spiritually evolve. How fortunate are we to be in a position of privilege that we have food and shelter. Be careful of how much you have fallen into the trap of MINE: MY house, MY car, MY holiday home. How much worth are you giving to your material possessions and how much is this driving your behaviour? Money, of course, has its value, and facilitates many wonderful things. However, we need to continually ask ourselves: How much is enough for me to lead a good life? I've gone through my own transition from earning a good salary to branching out on my own, and it has been a blessing to live more simply. Also, be attentive to your beliefs around money and your associated language when you talk about it. I am mindful to never make statements like, 'I can't do that because I don't have the money.' What you put out comes back tenfold! Come away from the mindset of lack, to one of 'I have everything I need.' Money is just one part of that. We can see that clearly in the visual representation of the balanced wellbeing fund. Money forms less than twenty per cent of it.

Watch the film *The Big Short* if you need more convincing about how money and ego can have dire consequences when left unchecked. The film brilliantly tells the story of the 2007/8 banking crisis. It is an excellent account, and it reminded me of what tense times these were. I was working for one of the big banks at the time and remember watching our share price drop from over $40 to below $5, which was just astonishing. We all sat around a colleague's computer and watched it in disbelief. How value can be lost in a matter of days, when the truth begins to unravel. This money obsession is very brain centric and, as such, is how, over the past few hundred years, we have chipped away at the beautiful connection and magnificence of our hearts. The heart knows, the heart feels and the heart loves. It is so much more powerful than the brain. And that is measurable, not just metaphorical.

Reflection on wealth

What is a comfortable monthly income for you?

What are your beliefs around money?

How do you speak about money? Does that reflect conditioned beliefs that no longer are helpful to you?

SELF-WORTH

Before saying something, a useful check-in is to ask yourself: "Is this helpful, or hurtful?" When we lash out at others, can we explore what is really going on from within ourselves?

When the 2008 Lehman's crisis precipitated the collapse of the global economy, rehabilitation centres for private clients who lost their jobs were full. In some severe and tragic cases, people committed suicide, as their self-worth had become so intricately tied to their financial earnings and status. They were unable to see beyond what life would look like without that big job, or title.

Paying attention to how you value yourself can help you see where limiting patterns and dialogue are manifesting. For me, a big part of knowing and feeling your worth is to build self-awareness. This is where meditation was the path I needed to truly connect with conscious awareness. I felt awareness in the body, not just residing in the head. This is not always an easy process or comfortable at all. But it is a path worth treading if we wish to liberate ourselves to live a truer life and switch on our inner awareness. The more we develop self-awareness, the more we see clearly what triggers us, and why those triggers are there. We can absolutely unlearn these reactions and unhelpful conditioning to heal the triggers. Over time, we learn to consciously respond to situations, conversations and plans, rather than react. Addictions creep in when we are not consciously responding. And, indeed, addictions are, in essence, a lack of self-love, where self-esteem and value have departed, or not had the nurturing terrain to grow.

Even when building a spiritual practise, we can fall into just doing it rather than really experiencing it. Regardless of whether you are sitting on the meditation cushion, coming to the yoga mat, or having an honest conversation with a loved one, do this from a place of true support to yourself. Listening is a big one here. And I mean listening to attend with presence, not listening in order to jump in with your response. There is quite a lot of spiritual bypassing, or even spiritual peacocking, that goes on, where people have created a veneer of that they 'think' is the right spiritual path. But that simply becomes just another distraction. Your spiritual practise will open your heart and help you come home.

To be 'in' the experience, we need to pay attention. And that is essentially becoming more self-aware and more deeply present. Avoidance is simply turning away from feeling. I know that one for sure. Part of the reason it took me years to heal from the demise of my longest relationship is because I got stuck in all the sadness, and developed a pattern of putting on a 'just carry on' face. Some experiences are indeed very painful and create deep emotional scars. These sufferings can be accrued through lifetimes. This is called Samskara in Sanskrit, or karmic scarring. It's a concept that we have been here before in a human body, through the experience of our soul. This can go a long way to help us understand our experiences better and surely allows a greater sense of expansiveness. What do we really know?

Stop thinking in linear time. Expand beyond the human construct of time, into a sense of limitlessness.

Reflection on Self-Worth

How much do you really love yourself ?

How do you express that in your day to day life and relationships?

How willing are you to value yourself and know yourself as fully as possible?

SUPPORT

'*Community is the guru of the future.*' A quote from master Buddhist teacher, Thich Nhat Hanh. We can change this to community is the guru of NOW. This support segment would apply to your personal and professional network, as well as the wider community that features in your day-to-day life. How can we help each other in day to day life to awaken our inner physician?

Under this piece of the wellbeing fund is your family, friends and relationships – both personal and professional.

Just think about how a sour look from a stranger can impact your whole day.

All of these components contribute to your health. There is no specific category in the wellbeing fund for 'health', because all of these facets make up your health and wellbeing. When we understand energy more coherently, we understand that all is vibration. Everything that exists in life operates under a vibration. So when we nurture all aspects of the wellbeing fund, we nurture the vibration level we each operate at. The higher this is, the more it will attract. This is the law of nature.

What vibration are you operating at? In turn, what vibration do you attract? Can you seek solutions in your world of dreams? What books do you choose? What films/plays/music/shows?

All your choices directly influence and reflect your energy field. How much are you paying attention to this subtle force? Do you find yourself just going through the motions, because you have checked out of being wholly alive?

Reflection on Support

Who makes your heart sing?

Who supports you honestly?

How discerning are you at choosing with whom you spend your time?

Does obligation rule your decisions, instead of your heart?

How does your energy feel after seeing certain people?

Dare you smile at a stranger? Do you fear connection? Why? What made you disconnect?

CHAPTER SEVEN

The power of the therapeutic rapport

"Excellent healthcare is best delivered by people who are themselves thriving and well."

I came across this phrase on the NHS Action for Wellbeing website. Super! I love the message it sends out. I very much agree that we — both the doctor and patient — all need to be as healthy as we can be, in order to be present in our experiences. This is what I mean by the power of the therapeutic rapport.

However, we have become massively hypnotised by a very drug centric health approach. This is a health system that is often now referred to as 'disease management' and is the very opposite of what truly serves public health. Our systems need to support us towards health and vitality and not just some low vibration disease management, dependent on chemicals and the publicly traded stock of Big Pharma. The degree to which each person is hypnotised is linked to their wakefulness. How aware are you of how to really help yourself? This is a key component we all must ask of ourselves and I very much encourage such self-reflection amongst the doctors and physicians, too. I appreciate it can be hugely triggering. We are asking ourselves to look at our stuff rather than deny it, based on what we have learned, been told, or what behaviour has been modelled to us through education. So many variables. This is why it can only work well with each person embracing who they are honestly. Then, collectively, we will be stronger, safer, and more trustworthy.

For patients to make the best choice for their treatment, they need all the options. This also shows how important patient awareness is. They need to ask questions and be in an active dialogue with their doctor and healthcare team. It is, absolutely, a conversation.

There is already a considerable movement within medical professionals towards a more integrated approach to health. Let me expand on what I mean by integrated: it means there are more tools available to this type of physician to help their patients. The wider system also supports this integrated approach, so it is cohesive, and less fractious and confusing. This will include excellent case taking, holding safe space for the patient and doing the work themselves, so they lead by example. They will also be able to advise on other avenues to explore for their health, such as yoga, physiotherapy, Reiki, bodywork and nutrition. The inaugural Yoga in Healthcare conference, held in February 2019, has started a very powerful conversation around integrating yoga into the NHS. This is vital for both staff and patients and has the potential to save billions in health costs.

All of our social systems that were put in place to help and support us have become the very things that are sabotaging our wellbeing. Health and education, political, economic and religious systems, all come with these enormous challenges and frustrations. They are, however, a wider reflection of collective consciousness and we all must keep focussed on believing in a better world, so we can make it happen through action and belief. Each one of us is responsible for that. How we show up matters. That is the therapeutic rapport. It cannot be one sided.

As a child, when I became sick and hospitalised in Dublin, a young doctor had to present my case to a fairly large medical audience. Before the presentation, I was wheeled down (not impressed that I had to sit in a wheelchair when I was capable of walking!) and he erratically, and in quite an anxious state, asked me hurried questions. I could absolutely feel his anxiety. His fear was palpable. When he came to present to the audience in the room, he was a bundle of nerves and got my age wrong, and bumbled out a muddled case history of my situation that certainly made no sense to me. If a child can't understand what you just said I thought, you've missed the mark. I just stayed quiet and felt for his state of panic.

It was an early insight into the psychology of some schools of medicine. That there can be such an emphasis on impressing peers and seniors, while disregarding of the patient, especially a child far away from home. Or, indeed, a lack of support for junior doctors. Where was the heart in this? There was no kindness or reassurance shown to me by him or, indeed, any other person in the room. I was a ten-year-old girl, sick and far from home, sitting there like a specimen. It was a horrible experience for me. It's possible that these early experiences set the tone for me understanding it was imperative I seek my own path on being well within myself. Thus, I am so appreciative to have encountered a kind and intuitive doctor like Professor Thompson during my early years in South Africa. Thank God for that powerful frame of reference. He was a true earth angel to me, setting me on a path to understanding how to help myself.

I spent three years studying the meaning of nutrition in a holistic sense. We learned about the foundations of bio-chemistry, anatomy and physiology, the details of macro and micro nutrients, as well as the major disease processes that can impact the different body systems. But we also learned to enquire, on a deeper level, into the health of our patients. Why were they self-sabotaging with their food choices? What was their belief around emotional health? How were they sleeping? What connections were there between eating certain foods and experiencing certain symptoms? How was their health as a child? What levels of stress were present and what was their body language?

Taking a good case history is absolutely key to understanding your patient. This is very much a required skill for any health practitioner and it comes from a combination of natural instinct and experience. Whilst a student at the College of Naturopathic Medicine in London, I took the case histories of my parents and sister during my first year of study. Whilst I knew these three people very well, by taking their individual cases I learned more about them than ever. You can learn so much from a one hour, in depth consultation with your patient. It is an intimate and considered experience, in a supportive and comfortable environment. Sadly, for many reasons, this approach is not much seen, or indeed, promoted in orthodox medical systems. Too much time pressure, too much paperwork, too much hierarchy. The list goes on. And the paradigm becomes more embedded. Nothing changes if we do not question it and be part of the change.

No nephrologist in our Western setting has asked me wider questions around my health. I am never asked about menstrual cycle, levels of stress in my life or how I sleep. It is all very linear and highly clinical. They look at labs, recommend drugs and ask standardised questions around peripheral oedema or breathlessness. So as long as we are aware of the limitations, we can work around them. But if we believe this traditional approach to be the only route to wellness, it likely won't be, especially with a chronic illness.

I remember hearing once something along the lines of; 'You can only take someone as far as you yourself have gone.' To me, as a holistic nutrition practitioner and yoga teacher, this really landed and certainly continues to motivate me to keep doing the inner work on myself. This means I can take others further, beyond where they first thought they could be. When I limit myself, I limit others. We are all mirrors. This is why what we do individually affects the whole collective. When you hold yourself back, you hold others back by clawing at the web of fear created by our current systems.

This is why there is always more research around health to read, more speakers to see and be inspired by, and scope for more experimentation with my own food and lifestyle choices. I am a risk taker and, alongside nutrition, am very happy to experiment on myself for the greater good. and to see how it feels and works for me. I get that not everyone will be this way and that's ok. Keep meeting yourself where you are at. Much of this shift and drive is now coming from the medical community; from doctors who are practicing with their eyes wide open and seeing the system patterns for what they are – and how they are not serving their patients.

How much inner work are the people who you look to for your healthcare doing? How enthusiastically and passionately does your doctor reach for his prescription pad? Do you leave your appointment feeling assured, empowered and listened to? Does your doctor look healthy and happy? These are just considerations to ponder. Of course, at the bare bones of it we are all in this human existence together and doctors are humans like anyone else. So I certainly don't wish for the message to be, 'doctors are this, patients are that'. We all oscillate, we all feel lost sometimes, we all feel empowered or disempowered in whatever we do. How can we collectively honour the therapeutic rapport together? How can we both take responsibility in this complex equation of exchange – where the formula relates to something as deeply personal as our own health, our own existence, our own care?

Holistic psychiatrist Dr Kelly Brogan speaks very clearly and honestly on this. She highlights that the levels of conflictive interest within the medical system are rarely addressed. We make assumptions that there are appropriate checks and balances in Government recommendations, which is not always the case. How much awareness are you prepared to tolerate? Once the lights have been switched on and shone down to see the murkiness, you can switch the lights off; but you will remember the murkiness you saw. Doctors are courted by pharma. We know this. They speak of it themselves. Pharma has its place, but when it starts to become a pattern of damaging and mindless prescribing, as a populace, we need to wake up. We need decisions that are based on truth and science. When there are more robust outcomes without pharma, why would you prescribe? It is not in the best interests of supporting your patient. The literature is there. Education for medical students needs to embrace this so they are better equipped for the next generation: to foster true health and turn around this epidemic of chronic disease. We must all be part of changing the tide.

I am not anti-pharma or anti vaccine. I don't believe in aligning myself with just one viewpoint and becoming fixated, as it is not helpful. I observe too many people at the mercy of their long time, conditioned beliefs, who get stuck defending something that they may not have fully explored. And I must of course remind myself that, over the course of my experience, some drugs have helped and been very necessary in my own life. Plus, the very fact that I rely on a medical machine to currently sustain my life. So, I must be balanced in my view and be fair, as much as possible. Justice can prevail for everyone, when each of us is fair. We do need ongoing dialogue, though, and for this to be more encouraged. I am 100 per cent pro-choice. To have true choice, you need to educate and inform yourself. You need to know there are always options, and know what these options are. I have noticed through my own experiences that there tends to be a lack of understanding of a patient's own expertise and knowledge.

For example, I studied nutritional medicine for three years in order to more deeply inform myself and to more effectively and safely help others. I attend regular Continual Professional Development (CPD) events to continue to build on my knowledge with some of the most progressive and cutting edge doctors in the world, and I also learn something new from every client I work with. My many years studying yoga has provided a very strong knowledge base, not only of my own body, but also the overall complexity of physiology and anatomy of the body and of the soul. I guess it's wise to never assume you're the cleverest or most knowledgeable person in the room – in a patient/doctor scenario, it's often assumed by the doctor that they know best. Is this instilled in medical school? Are doctors taught to believe they know better and are not to be questioned? This pattern does not make the medic an unpleasant person, it just reflects the current circumstance of training, as well as their lack of understanding of the bigger picture. When I had my catheter fitted, my brilliant nurse talked through the procedure, as two paramedics had asked my permission to attend and observe. The nurse explained to them that the insertion was going beneath the greater omentum, which is the apron like adipose tissue layer covering the front trunk of the body. I understood perfectly what this was, but the nurse apologised to me for the technical language. This is not a reflection of bad form, it is just an assumption made that the patient doesn't know much. And I apply that to myself too! So, when I meet a new patient or client for the first time, I also have to understand how much they know about themselves. It has to be an exchange without assumption. Conversely, I need to remember I have the gift of many years of study and experience and that sometimes my lovely, intelligent, new clients are simply coming to me for guidance – as they openly admit their nutritional awareness is minimal. This includes doctors who are also my patients, and I love that. Each day we plant a seed to meet ourselves where we are at, through the turbulence and uncertainty that is part of the flow of life. But we can also truly meet others where they are at, without judgment. Remember to be fair and open minded. And I am absolutely saying this to myself too!

Patients would naturally diverge from conventional medicine when they knew all the options. So, it all comes down to EDUCATION!

The wonder of the Social Prescribing movement

In February 2018, when my good friend Katie forwarded me an invitation to a 'Social Prescribing' meeting, I was intrigued, not having heard the term before. The local vicar hosted the meeting in the vicarage, encouraging his church to be a light in the community, rather than something only available to those with certain beliefs. There was quite a collection of people who gathered for this meeting, including GPs and Practice Managers, a fitness instructor and a choir leader. Together, we embarked on a discussion around community engagement. Essentially, the social prescribing movement aims to facilitate more access to activities and support within the community. So, for example, GPs can signpost their patients towards specific community endeavours, ranging from yoga and meditation, to debt advice. This encourages the patient to take action and understand what is available to help them. My heart was singing loudly during this meeting. It was the morning after I had given my first local inspirational speaking talk, and I was on fire from within with passion and hope. I was so heartened – especially after having had many moments of deep frustration over the years with the health system. I was intent on discovering ways I could help. This opportunity was exactly that. We heard how two of the people from the movement had got in front of Simon Stevens, the Chief Executive of NHS England, and his leadership team, to explain what this was about. Where we start to make real differences is by truly helping each other and leaning into the support of community. And what a wonderful way to also empower people to awaken their inner physician. As a result of this one meeting, I became the yoga teacher for two local community classes, where my rate was funded and the classes were free to the community. And I get so much from teaching these classes. The class attendance is far more diverse than one might see in a pricey yoga studio. I very much believe that the truth of yoga should be available to all. When you help people connect more with the simplicity of their breath, and encourage a safe space for each person to arrive and do the inner engineering they need in a community setting, it is so powerful. This also means that a local group of people are coming together so, especially if there is social isolation, this is another avenue into feeling part of a group; a reminder that we are all so much more connected than our minds can ever believe.

One-to-one counselling and mindfulness are also being brought to the community under this umbrella. I have visions of bringing nutrition to this as well, especially to help GPs develop their nutritional knowledge. There is so much to be excited about. It's all up for change and although NHS bureaucracy means this integrated approach now being explored is not without challenge, together we can make these changes and implement them safely, smoothly and effectively. It truly is all possible.

Working one-to-one with people

The intensity of working one-to-one with people can bring up all sorts of emotions and this will absolutely have a bearing on the quality of the therapeutic rapport. Especially when working with how people feel. Yoga helps you be in your body and begin the internal inquiry of 'What's really going on here? How am I, really? Can I even face these questions?' It provides the space for reflection, for stillness. To explore in a safe and supported environment, and then integrate what you experience on the mat into the daily fabric of your life. Given this context, working one-to-one with all kinds of people requires deep self-awareness and clear boundaries on what is yours and what is not.

How do we learn what these boundaries are? I have learned this through various life experiences, such as in a college environment, observing myself at my own regular hospital and doctor appointments, and all my self-exploration through yoga, shamanism and meditation. I've been my inner alchemist. I've also learned, the hard way, what not to do. Boundaries can become blurred. People become co-dependent. This is not healthy for either side in a professional, or in a personal, context.

There has to be an improved patient understanding that the practitioner (be it a doctor or any other kind of therapist) cannot hold all the answers for you. Your willingness to share honestly will be reflected in their response. Help them understand you. Let them take a brilliant case history – your answers and engagement depend on that. If you arrive skeptical and untrusting, you are more likely to leave skeptical and untrusting. Set the tone.

And what a sense of empowerment comes from taking action and having an understanding of what is happening to you. When you raise your own vibration through action and understanding, it percolates and raises the vibration for people in your circle. That's how we shift collective consciousness. We are all responsible for what becomes the cosmic heart.

When fear is instilled into the patient by a doctor – who says, for example, 'if you don't do/take this, this will happen' – this is, in part, a projection of their own fears. When choices are fear based, they are far less likely to be in our best interests, or to serve us well. I do understand there is the other side to this: if a patient is being difficult, refusing bluntly to listen, or becoming abusive, for example. I understand when speaking bluntly might be necessary for the doctor to make their point. But if we created a clear code of expected behaviours from one another, this bluntness might then not be required from either side. It's a bit like those signs you see in a lot of public services - on transport, or in a GP waiting room - about not behaving in an abusive manner towards the staff. Could we change this message to reflect that we all must respect each other? This would come across as more caring and take account of both sides, rather than feeling quite disturbed when we read that sign. It is terrible to think that staff might be regularly at risk of abuse or attack. Those people who do become violent or abusive are letting the whole system down, but of course there will also be a deeper basis for their behaviour. This is a highly complex area when, for example, the issue is substance abuse. Addicts are far less likely to take responsibility and, sadly, our modern society is perfused with all sorts of addiction. We all have elements of this to some extent, so this is where ongoing self-exploration becomes so important.

During my hospital stay in Spring 2016, preparing to be discharged, one of the senior registrars came by on his rounds. I had heard him in the previous room speaking quite loudly and condescendingly to a male patient, who was clearly at the point of coming to terms with losing his own kidney function, and being prepared for haemodialysis. Perhaps the doctor felt he needed to speak bluntly in order to be understood, but to me it came across as a very harsh, even cruel, tone. I felt for the man and it also made me ask of myself, how on earth did I cope with processing all of that at just fourteen years old?

This doctor was then preparing to come into my room, so he was masking up (as I was at risk of infection at this point). It's funny how, in a hospital environment, some medical staff act as if the patient cannot hear; that somehow, because they are unwell, they have lost their ability to hear, or have suddenly become a bit thick. For me, because I was in such a great space within myself and deeply present, I was also highly sensitive to other people's energy. I could hear the doctor outside my room, asking his two female colleagues - who both came across as very keen to impress this man - my name. They did not once glance my way - namely, in the direction of the actual patient. He was struggling to get the pronunciation of my name, a common issue for people as it's Irish. It would have been much less stressful for all involved if he'd just come in, introduced himself and simply asked, how do you pronounce your name? Instead, he was getting increasingly agitated and ended up just stating, "I still didn't get the name," before coming in. All this right outside where I was – so clearly within earshot. This was revealing to me about his state: frenetic, tense, rushed, and clearly used to younger staff falling at his feet, or responding to his demands. I did feel like saying to him; "Dude, sit yourself down and let yourself relax, you're going to give yourself a heart attack!" However, that was not my role in that context and so I calmly asked the questions I had. I wanted to know how my CRP level was doing, as it had been so high on admittance. CRP stands for C-Reactive Protein and is a helpful marker for inflammation. Mine had been through the roof, after never having previously been an issue. A healthy CRP is below 2. Mine was seriously elevated at over 100. He shouted out the door, "Can I get a trend on the CRP?" Jesus! I thought. Where are we? On the trading floor of the Chicago Mercantile Exchange?! In response to all the questions I had about some of the meds I had been prescribed, he said, "Give us six months to sort things out."

Fair enough, I thought. I could see his point. But I said to myself, and felt it inside, that in six months I'd be flying and not worrying about meds. I made my own decisions and it all worked out fine. That is the power of seeking counsel from your inner physician.

I understood we were all adapting to a new chapter. However, I also knew inside that the next six months were a time for me to continue the inner alchemy. That would be where the magic I was already experiencing would happen, with such a swift recovery and jubilant mood. One of the points I made to this doctor was that I did not want to be on a proton pump inhibitor for the long term. This is a class of drugs that suppresses stomach acid production and is not good news for much longer than two or three weeks. I had understood it had been prescribed on admittance because when urea levels are so high, there can be a risk of internal bleeding. My steroid dose had also been doubled from the 5 mg maintenance dose to 10 mg, which I was keen to begin to tail off again. I'm pleased to say now I am fully off the steroids, which my consultant suggested some months later – and I was thrilled to comply. This was a window to rest my body from any immune-suppression protocol. I was very pleased to hear this, as I'd been given the impression that I had to stay on a maintenance dose of steroids due to the risk of the kidney rejecting, which could result in serious infection and it having to be removed. I also ceased the proton pump inhibitor shortly after coming out of hospital of my own accord, and fed that back during my appointments in the renal unit. If I did not question this, or had not had my own knowledge around this drug, I would probably still be taking it and wreaking more damage internally. This class of drugs is now emerging as having many undesirable side effects, including compromised immunity, in part because stomach acid is a key line of defence against potential incoming invaders to the body. Stomach acid is also needed for effective protein assimilation, as well as healthy iron absorption. This, I fear, happens way too often. People are prescribed something without fully understanding what it's for, how it's working or, indeed, if it is necessary, or helpful. And without understanding that there are other ways they can heal the issue, without pill popping.

But back to the hospital doctor. As he left the room, I heard him say: 'She had a lot of questions'.

For the sake of clarity, I do still have Kenny kidney in my body and whilst in terms of removing metabolic waste he's only minimally performing. He does, however, still produce urine which is wonderful. It means I am not restricted on fluid intake, which had been enormously challenging. I still have about eight per cent function, which is definitely helpful in light of how much kidneys do.

My surrender meant my hospital experience was a good one. I didn't worry, and I took all the new information in about PD with great awareness. I did note, however, that no-one really acknowledged that I had just gone through a major life event and lost my transplant kidney function. None of the nurses on the ward acknowledged it, and neither did the pharmacists. There was a renal counsellor who did – a lovely role the unit has funded which I applaud but, in my view, compassion must not be isolated to that role alone. The only person who did say, 'I'm sorry' when I told her why I was there, was a delightful young female paramedic, who was doing a rotation on the unit. I'm sure she is a marvellous addition to the ambulance service. She was one of the paramedics who asked my permission to come and observe the catheter fitting, and I was fully supportive of this as she was so enthusiastic. She stepped in to hold my hand during the procedure at one point, when the other nurse was occupied. I deeply appreciated such support.

There was an otherwise general feeling on the ward that the staff were just getting on with things, with the communication lines running between each of them and the patient largely disregarded. For example, during one nurse handover, they did not even acknowledge me in the bed while they discussed me. The day after I had had the catheter fitted was also after that long 12-hour dialysis session, and it was very painful for me to get up. I expressed this to the nurse in my room at the time, who said, "You can just walk to the toilet." No, I really couldn't. I felt very fragile in this moment and some big fat tears began to roll down my face, as I just needed a helping hand. She did go and get a commode at that point, having sensed my upset, but it was tough and was the first time I'd had a bit of a cry in hospital. I find this a bizarre way to behave. Again, I don't know what drives this. Do they wish to have the least patient involvement possible? Is there a belief that it is an easier option and a more efficient way to work? I'm not cross about this, I am merely observing it, based on my own experience.

This does, however, make a good conversation all the more valuable when it happens. So, when one of the female senior consultants explained to me there was a nodule on my lung, so they were going to send me for a full CAT scan, this could have been alarming. However, she went on to say, in a very kind and confident manner, that she wasn't worried about it and that it was most likely due to the chest sepsis. I was greatly relieved by this exchange, as I did have a fleeting thought that I wasn't sure I'd cope with what was already going on – and then a tumour! However, my inner voice and instincts told me it was nothing to worry about, and I believe that was reflected in what the doctor had communicated to me. There is always a deeper flow of energetic communication happening.

I actually did not have that confirmed for some days and, in the meantime, a less experienced younger doctor came and spoke to me as if I was of limited intellect. Almost shouting this at me, they said the scan was being done because the nodule could be malignant due to the immuno-suppression drugs, which increase this risk. Having already had the earlier conversation about this with the more experienced doctor, reconciling my concerns, I found this tone and language completely inappropriate. But I just observed it, realising it was important for me to trust my instincts and not be bothered by what this second doctor had said. What makes one doctor relay information kindly, but still with the same content, versus another who scaremongers and massively generalises, ignoring the context of the patient? Did they think I did not already know the risks involved with the immuno-suppression medications, and need such information thrown at me during a vulnerable time? Again, we have to ask what drives this rather base behaviour. Is it a feeling of superiority? Were they influenced in medical school, is it a conditioned belief from their own family or is it just lack of self-awareness? Probably a combination of all those things. Given the hours she was working too, she was probably exhausted. And in some way, I imagine if a doctor has a certain level of anxiety to deal with within themselves, this might make them a bit nervous and clumsy in how they relay information. Lucky for me I was able to consider all aspects, because I was in such a calm state and could see the bigger picture. If not, I might have fretted hugely and severely hindered my recovery. It transpired the nodule was harmless and in keeping with the chest sepsis, although I only discovered this from reading my discharge letter. I am incredibly grateful to be able to discern these behaviours as projections of people's own personalities and beliefs, rather than absorb them and start to believe them for myself. This is so key. Don't let in the things that other people say, if it really doesn't feel right to you. So many patients become their diagnosis and believe all that is told to them, without the necessary application of ongoing discernment. This is why the conscious spiritual excavation is so important. It becomes a combination of surrender and will. You start to know when to choose surrender and let it go, and when to choose the will to challenge. Nothing changes if things are not challenged: the culture just becomes more deeply embedded.

Coming back to the renal counsellor, I had never known this was available or asked for it, but it seemed it was routine for a counsellor to come and see in-patients on the renal ward. She was a lovely lady, who came and stood in my doorway a couple of days after I had been admitted, and introduced herself. She was absolutely delightful, and it was so comforting to have someone there, in that capacity, to hold safe space. She also had a keen interest in yoga, so we talked about that. She came to see me three times during my one week stay. Support always comes, it really does. I remember saying to her how I was doing very well and that I was waiting for the meltdown to come. It never came. And I realise there was no need for a meltdown, because of the journey I had taken in the preceding years. I can only surmise on how I might have been had I still been working a hectic job in banking, and not exploring the deeper aspects of being human. I might have fallen into a deep depression and felt very sorry for myself. However, I was so replete with joy and surrender, I worried not at all.

My best friend and her husband came to the rescue and picked me up from hospital to take me home after this hospital stint, in Spring 2016. Back to my dear house in the woods. My home. My haven. My sanctuary. Wherever I am in the world, I always love returning here. As we pulled up, there were two magpies sitting on the roof. Magpies have become one of my animal totems in recent years. With my burgeoning interest in shamanic practise and alchemy, I have come to understand the deep wisdom all of nature holds, and how it speaks to us through its form. That day it was saying, 'Welcome home, Ciara'. I felt so happy and comforted.

Once I was alone, I remember standing in front of my mirror in the lounge and looking deep into my own face. I had shape shifted. In that moment, I could see it so clearly. Something had lifted off me energetically. My nose had changed shape. It was slimmer. My California cousin, Lisa, was the only one who noticed this a few days later when she visited. She is very intuitive and I have learned a lot from her over the years, travelled to many far flung and exciting places together, and had deep and long conversations about the human experience with her.

"You have a new nose!" she exclaimed. "I know," I smiled back, as I could feel it represented such a profound internal shift.

It's uplifting to remember this was my first in-patient hospitalisation since 1998, when I'd had to be re-admitted to Oxford to have a second operation to replace the necrotic donor ureter. So, I had been a very well person for many years. I'd had a one-day outpatient experience several years previously for the excision of one of my para-thyroid glands. This came about as I had slightly elevated calcium levels in my blood, along with slightly elevated para-thyroid hormone levels. In hindsight, I would perhaps not have had this surgery, especially as afterwards, when it did not really resolve the issue, the surgeon said, "Well your calcium wasn't that high." That would have been a useful comment to take on board before the surgery. I just did not have enough of my own skills at that time to say, 'actually, I'm not going to have that surgery.' Sorry, body, to have put you through that. If I knew what I know now and understood the context better, I would have appreciated that the surgery was likely not necessary.

Now I am listed within the current transplant pool, so I trust the right kidney will come up if that is the route I am meant to take. I also pay great attention to looking after myself whilst on PD. The visions I have for myself is wellness and light, and that means being strong and healthy on all levels. I don't like to describe it as, 'I am waiting for a kidney.' I'm not waiting for something to happen to live my life. I live my life as fully as possible, always. Sometimes that means weeping as if my heart is breaking, sometimes that means smiling hugely as if I am a dog in a car with its head lolling out the window – unbound delight. And I continue to dwell in all possibilities. The capacity to heal is infinite. There is so much already that I have healed from. I apply no limits to what is infinitely possible. And that is a very hopeful way to live.

In preparation for being listed for another kidney, there were a series of steps required. Part of this approved protocol was meeting one of the surgeons. This meeting was scheduled for me when my first transplant was still functioning sufficiently to not require dialysis, and the intention had been to pre-emptively be listed and for a kidney to come up before dialysis was needed. This is a tricky timeline to manage, as no-one knows how long a kidney will keep going. So I went off to meet the surgeon, endeavouring to keep an open mind, but still quite trepidatious. I intended the meeting to be fruitful and useful. Setting intentions for events is a highly effective, positive visualisation to give yourself.

I sat waiting ahead of my appointment, and the next thing a lady in a wheelchair emerged from the consulting room, deeply distressed and shouting, very loudly, "He can keep his kidney!" She was clearly referring to the surgeon who she had just had the appointment with. And I was up next!

Oh Jesus. Here I am, wanting to have a calm experience – and this poor woman has evidently not had the best dialogue with the surgeon. It was then more difficult for me to envisage a positive experience. I did see the irony in the situation. I was so intent on manifesting a positive experience for myself. It is rare to see patients shouting like that in hospital. When it does happen, it is not fun. It's raw and almost too intimate to witness as an outsider.

So I braced myself as my name was called. This was the first time we were meeting and these meetings can feel heavily weighted, as part of you feels that if this person does not want to recommend you for transplant, it could have devastating consequences. Let me be heard, let me be understood. Let me speak truthfully and calmly.

There was a sense of tension in the air following what must have been a tough conversation with the previous woman, but he made no reference to it. The great unsaid lingered and I sat down, feeling slightly wide eyed. We chatted and I felt it necessary to raise my experience of coming off all medication for a number of years. Although I initiated this point, I knew that he would doubtless have the information on file, as it is so unusual. He was quite flippant in his response, something along the lines of, 'What did you do that for?' I sensed this conversation was going to become more tense and I was getting more internally upset, so I just said, "Look, I don't want to come out of here totally stressed out."

I went on to flex some intellectual muscle, as my friend Katie says, around the facts. I explained I had tailed off immuno-suppression over many, many years, very slowly and carefully, monitoring my kidney function all the while. This actually showed an improvement, my blood pressure was perfect and I was then asked by the hospital to participate in the tolerance studies. I said I was quite sure these would yield more important information around transplant medication, and a greater understanding around why some people can 'tolerate' the transplanted organ, whereas others reject their organs quite quickly without medication. I wanted to be clear on the sequence of events and demonstrate I did this from a responsible place of deep intuition, not as a self-saboteur or ignoramus. Being made to feel like I had deliberately precipitated a decline in my precious transplant was deeply hurtful. There are junctures in life, during these potentially difficult conversations, where we must fill in the gaps, or clarify correctly. Often, people get too nervous in these situations, which I utterly empathise with, yet we must still be brave enough to have the best conversation we can in our own best interests. And this is not easy.

An interesting comment the surgeon also made was: "You could have had a 30-year kidney." This, again, hurt. Whoever knows what may, or may not, have been. Would my kidney still be going now if I hadn't tailed off the drugs completely? I just don't know. No-one does. Correlation does not prove causation. And a 30-year kidney is rare, especially from a cadaveric unrelated donor. Regardless, the inflammatory cascade, once triggered, can be incredibly difficult to hold back, or reverse, once the complement substance starts to lay down. This can happen, and often does happen, when still on immuno-suppression medication, and is the big question in transplantation around the shelf life of organs. I don't have the answers. I know I did what felt right for me and that it was of great benefit to me in the years I had been on mono-therapy, and then on no drugs.

I also provided more content for the ongoing research around tolerance. As the lead nephrologist on the tolerance studies at Guys said on this topic: "We are using cannon balls to kill flies." The impact of heavy duty drugs matters.

I am fortunate in that I understand there are ways to manage the side effects of the drugs through healthy lifestyle, dietary choices and deep self-enquiry. Yet still, it is not the perfect answer, and more research is needed in the area of personalised drug protocol for each individual.

In fairness, the surgeon did acknowledge my contribution to the tolerance research, and said this outcome could have happened anyway. I did feel that at nearly 20 years with this first transplant I'd had, on reflection, a very good innings, and wanted to be grateful and acknowledging of that. Putting an expectation onto me to have a 30- year kidney was quite considerable, yet it did mirror what I always initially thought: I never put a shelf life on Kenny kidney. I always viewed him as my partner for life, which I feel was an important contributor to the subsequent longevity I had with him. I wasn't thinking all the time, 'When will this reject?' Mindset matters.

Another requirement before being listed is to attend a seminar presented by the transplant team. This includes a surgeon, a transplant co-ordinator, a nurse and a pharmacist. My friend kindly offered to come with me, so off we went. This was very much a box ticking exercise and, given I have already been through the experience of having a kidney transplant, there was nothing new for me to hear. These kinds of events were not on offer when I was originally listed; all I had to do then was meet the head professor in Oxford, who was a lovely man. I went to that meeting with Parley, so it was intimate and unthreatening. This wider event in London, which had about another twenty patients and one or two family members with each of them, was useful to a point, but also quite terrifying for those who had no experience of this. I could tell by the odd gasp or muttering as the presentation went on that it was a lot to take in for people unfamiliar with it. I guess that makes it in some part helpful, but in some part instills more fear. It could actually massively trigger some people, leaving them feeling isolated and distressed.

Despite my initial meeting with the surgeon feeling quite charged, I received a letter some weeks later where he recommended me as a good candidate for transplant. It was extremely well written and demonstrated that he had totally understood the situation – although it might not have felt like it during the appointment. I do recall him saying at one stage in the meeting: "Well, you're a completely different person now." I felt this was astute of him. I had assured him my intention was certainly not to come off all meds again. Given my experience, I would not do that now, but this does not mean I am regretful of my decision to cease the drugs at the time. I make choices to enhance and support my health, based significantly on how it makes me feel intuitively, not the opposite. I will, however, continue to be interested in the tolerance research, and

to keep an open mind around all the possibilities. I will also wish to be
on the lowest meds possible and on a regime that makes sense to me.
This, I know, will of course have to be an ongoing dialogue. Life is fluid,
always changing. And I also keep an open mind and interest in regenerative
medicine. Can my kidney damage be reversed through regeneration and
visualisation techniques? Can stem cell research help here? I really don't
rule anything out, because I am interested. The field of potentiality is
vast. I know how healing my body has happened on a multitude of levels
already in this lifetime. I remain curious for myself, and for others, who
are to experience this journey. I embrace my inner pioneer, as this is not
just about me, this is about us as a collective. Increasingly, I come across
patients who have had severe kidney damage diagnosed and are having
looming conversations with doctors around the next steps of dialysis
and transplantation. Many of these people then went away and informed
themselves before choosing another way to wellness. Kidney tissue
does regenerate. To say it does not is an untruth. The biological imprint
responds absolutely to our input, our foods, our thoughts, our sleep.
Everything influences everything, all of the time, so we do not need to
get stuck. When this happens, it is inevitably the mind that is grasping us
in fear. We are back in that evolutionary negative bias and going in circles,
trying to figure it out. When we drop that and come into the felt awareness
of the body, magic really can ensue. Remember, healing happens in many
forms. It might not be how you expect. Always keep an open mind.

It is useful to consider the health practitioners in your life and how they
do, or do not, inspire you to initiate change. What is their body language?
How do you feel after seeing them? How long did you have to wait? Was
any delay acknowledged and an apology offered? How long was your
appointment? As a practitioner, being understood is one the most powerful
things you can offer a patient in front of you. What is their choice of
vocabulary? Can you be alert to their conditioning – namely, what has
influenced their health and why they do what they do? So it does not, in

turn, become a dangerous influence on you. For both, this is about tuning in, being present.

I was told by one of the doctors about a man who never turned up, as he had a phobia of hospital appointments. I wondered if he just felt it was too stressful and he'd rather just be living his life. I can understand that to a point but, for me, I also know the importance of staying informed about what's going on. It is a great strength to be able to extrapolate the relevant and valuable information for yourself from these hospital appointments.

Do you feel safe, heard and understood in your dialogue with your health practitioner? And I mean all types of practitioner - from doctor to nurse, to physiotherapist to massage therapist. All of the one-to-one interactions you have in relation to your wellbeing. Can you take stock of your life on a regular basis? Being bone crushingly honest with yourself so, at the moment of your death, there are no regrets, just a giant beam of a smile and a thought: 'Wow, what an amazing journey.'

Because we are all responsible for our own experiences, in terms of how we respond in the moment. I don't mean we are responsible for bad things that happen to us; often, something happens in our childhood that sows the seed of pain and gets tucked away into the tissues. But collectively, it matters hugely how we navigate our personal circumstances and that we feel courageous enough to explore these darker sufferings. We open the sense doors and explore that way, not through the looping of the mind. We are influencing the entire matrix – how we vibrate affects how others feel. Through a spiritual practise we also learn to not judge anything as 'good' or 'bad' - it just is.

The incredibly fractured and disjointed health system leads to a broken belief that body systems are separate. They are not. Your whole body is an entire communication network. Nothing is intended to work in isolation.

That is the beauty and magnificence of the innate wisdom of the human body. A creation of nature that is infinitely wise.

In this fast-paced modern world, it is also incredibly helpful to have access to your healthcare team. For example, I have certain email addresses of the doctors and nurses in the renal unit that look after me, and it has become increasingly normal to have this level of contact in such a technological age. In my opinion, it harnesses efficiency, which can be difficult to achieve and foster in a large organisation, especially a public service. Of course, it's important to use this contact with care and respect, and I only send emails when it's necessary. This person-to-person interaction helps lessen the sense of feeling like a statistic, and more like a real person. Human to human.

What is the therapeutic rapport with yourself? How do you run your own internal dialogue? Honestly begin to ask yourself what are the blocks to your own healing, and how you can heal. What feels possible for you. Think about the role and power you give to your doctor: do you allow your doctor to be a block to your healing, or provide a cascade and catalyst for hope and action? What's the potential fallout for you after a hospital or doctor's appointment, and how does that manifest? Consider the potency of what is said in a therapeutic context.

How you manage your own internal dialogue matters. Self-reassurance can be really nurturing and calming. When I came out of hospital after nearly losing my life in 2016, following my chest infection and resulting health crisis, my breathing was quite laboured. I live in a hilly part of London and am a big walker. I recall walking up one of the hills and it was tough, but I just reassured myself, saying: 'It's ok. You can do this. One step at a time. You're amazing. You're doing so well.' And I really meant it for myself. It made me feel wonderfully calm and supported from within.

When things were initially starting to unravel in terms of kidney function in my transplant kidney, I found the hospital appointments very difficult, partly because often I presented such a calm exterior, asked questions, and showed little emotion. However, beneath this was turbulence. Great, churning turbulence. And I started a routine of calling Marley after these appointments, where I would cry and cry to her. Sobbing. I needed an outlet and my poor mother was the receiver. After a certain amount of weeks passing in this pattern, I had to check myself. No Ciara, your poor mother cannot be the ongoing receiver of these big emotional releases, although I am hugely grateful for her being there in that way for me. She kindly said to me during one of these phone calls, "You need to find a better way to handle these appointments." And she was absolutely right. And so, I dived into the turbulence. This was the only way to resolve it. Unburden yourself from the jaws of your past and the anxious anticipation of what's to come. This is what it means to come out of your shadow and see your shadow then for what it is.

I had to begin to unpick all of it. I had to watch the past like a movie reel of experience, scene by scene, from my teenage kidney failure, to haemodialysis, to transplant. I imagined the death of my dear donor, him lying on the operating table and his organs being harvested, before one of his precious kidneys was grafted into me. I imagined him as a little boy and all the hopes he had for himself. He was living his life and I, mine – and then a moment in time brought us the closest we could come; a piece of his body becoming mine. I supported myself with meditations, a lot of crying, and looking my fears right in the face. So close. I am so humbled by all of this. To have the opportunity to dive into the turbulence, to understand myself better, to acknowledge all the physical and emotional experiences this body has been through from the tender age of just 4 years old. And this helped me to develop such self compassion, which I realised I had not allowed myself to feel. I had simply kept going, achieving, learning, striving. What a gift to feel this deeply. What a gift. As writer, healer and metaphysician, Louise Hay says, "If you can feel, you can heal." I understand this viscerally now, and I am still discovering and remain ever curious. There is such beauty waiting to be revealed to us inside our pain.

We must take courage to go into the pain. We can only come through it by feeling it.

I remember experiencing myself, in my own body and mind, what it is to truly be the observer of my situation. 'Become the observer' is widely referenced in the yoga tradition. I was in a doctor's appointment and I just felt it drop in. Ah! Here I am, in this chair, having this conversation – and it's all ok. I am the compassionate observer, rather than the scared participant. It was extremely comforting and liberating at the same time. A relief. It was a transient feeling, however, which is why each day is a commitment to remain in your truth and present to your experience. The more one practises this, the more natural it feels.

There is a fine balance of feeling your feelings – and being willing and able to take action. So don't get stuck for too long in a certain emotion – move through it. You need to alchemically burn through the old emotions and truly transform. That is the phoenix rising from the ashes that have burned and released. How can you precipitate your own rescue mission? What can be turned around and what can be let go?

It's also fascinating to stay present, as much as possible, to our responses to what doctors say to us. I remember one appointment in 2013, when we were discussing the initial recommendation for me to have a kidney biopsy. This comes with all sorts of risk, including, very rarely an unstoppable bleed that could result in loss of the kidney altogether. I asked what the risks were and the doctor's response was, "It's operator dependent." The harsh reality is mistakes happen in medicine and they happen a lot. Many factors tie into this – a momentary lapse in concentration, a communication error, lack of experience, or fatigue. I did agree to proceed with the biopsy, because after this conversation it was my understanding it would yield a clear answer to why I was unwell. I was never told it might not give me this answer. So even after this risky procedure, I still didn't know if it was rejection, a reoccurrence of the nephritis I'd developed as a child, or a reaction to resuming the immuno-suppression medications – all of which were possibilities.

For the first kidney biopsy, which I wasn't very keen to go ahead with, Marley came to stay with me. Although this is now a daytime procedure, you have to lie flat for six hours afterwards and have someone at home with you during the night, in case of a later bleed. I sent her off to a cafe and told her to come back much later. They were well organised with the preparations, and I started talking to a younger doctor who was there. She did seem quite skittish and went on to read out all the risks of the procedure. She rounded it off by loudly stating, "…and then there's risk of death. Some people have died from a biopsy. I have to tell you that." Ok, so can we please take a view here on what is actually useful for me to hear! I'd already been given the form to sign, so I did not need this rather blatant review of the risks. It was such a climactic ending, which reverberated around the room, while I was having my observations taken by a nurse. So now, quite early in the morning, I'm feeling quite sensitive about it all.

She further worried me by telling me she might be doing the biopsy herself and that she'd never done a biopsy on a transplant kidney before! She did say that a more senior consultant was on his way and would likely be doing it. And, thankfully, in he walked. And as soon as I saw him, I felt immediately peaceful. That is how powerful a person's calm presence is – and this is a person I had never before met, or heard about. He came and sat on the bed, right by me, and asked to examine my graft site. As it became very clear he would be doing the biopsy, I was silently giving huge thanks. He talked me through the procedure, and then became quite animated when it was revealed I was one of the patients who had ceased all immuno-suppression meds. He said to me, "Are you a risk taker?" I answered no, but went on to add that I worked in Credit Risk, and hence was aware of what a risk assessment looked like. We both smiled and agreed this was quite ironic. In truth, I am a risk taker. Goodness, what is life without risk? We die in our comfort zone. It is also true to say my experience in banking taught me, when lending to wealthy private individuals, through rather complex financial structures, one's own instinct about a person counts hugely. So say I would present a credit lending case to the senior credit committee, someone might ask, 'Well, Ciara, what's your view having met the client?' That matters. At the end of the day, in any scenario, your gut instinct about a person matters. In a credit lending environment, the worse-case scenario is the client gets into financial difficulty and struggles to honour their debt payments. This is where having a good relationship and good judgement is so helpful when it comes to working out a solution for a bad debt. And I know this from experience, as the banks were flush with bad debts after the 2008 meltdown. You need the art of negotiation and understanding, and I think this also applies to the doctor/patient rapport. This doctor had an extremely calm and kind demeanour, was genuinely interested, and not judgemental of my history. His view was that I would likely need to resume immuno-suppression. Bear in mind, weeks were passing whilst decisions were being made on what to do. Interestingly, my kidney function did improve and almost normalise back to previous levels after I went on to resume the medications. Whilst on the surface I was very happy about that, something didn't feel right within me. It was almost as if I was being told there was more to do, there was more to feel, and this episode wasn't at an end. At a friend's wedding a few weeks later I felt dreadful. I had developed horrendous menstrual pains upon resumption of the drugs, and had to go to bed just after the ceremony in one of the guest bedrooms. After a few hours of sleep, I emerged after doing a big poo, feeling much improved. However, at my next clinic appointment, the subsequent lab results showed things had again spiralled. This was what I had been feeling, and not just physically: a sense that there was more depth to come from this experience, and more to unravel within myself.

After the kidney function showed it had again worsened, this was when my doctor called me and said that a second biopsy was necessary. I said I'd have to think about it, as by this point it was all becoming a bit too much. I had also booked a weekend away with Marley to go to Barcelona. After some thought, I figured that this would provide more clarity, as my doctor had also said at this point, "The drugs seem to be making things worse," which made me more confused again. I called her back and said I would proceed, but it would have to be the following week after Barcelona. I also asked if the doctor who did my first biopsy would do this one, too. She said she would ask him and within half an hour called me back to say she'd spoken to him, and he would absolutely do that for me. I greatly appreciated this, and it also goes to show that our needs and wishes in this context can be met. People understand. When he came to chat to me ahead of performing the second biopsy, he had the consent form for me to sign and I said, "I'll just sign it," without him listing the risks for me. He fully understood, saying, "Ah, you don't want me to do my speech, no problem." Again, understanding can come from people.

What education is there around bedside manner and effective communication during a medical degree? I don't know. And I imagine, too, that this will vary in different colleges, and vary culturally between countries. There is considerable conditioning around society's belief about the role of doctors: this reverence of medics and the idea that what the doctor says is absolute. It is not. Sometimes it is wonderful and useful advice, sometimes it is damaging. There are so many variables.

How much expectation do you put in your doctor to feed you all the answers and solutions? Do you realise you may give your power away in this process if the expectation is all on them? This is co-dependency. How much influence is it right to assign to one person in this context? How outdated is this context? Who challenges it within the system?

First, do no harm. This is one of the pillars of naturopathic medicine. The wonderful neuro-surgeon Henry Marsh's first book, titled Do No Harm, provides such a marvellously honest and brave account of his experiences in brain surgery. I'm so pleased Marley passed this book onto me, as these kinds of honest stories speak to our humanity, the immense pressure some medics are under, and how they navigate it. And it is important to remember that doctors and surgeons are human and fallible and that they, too, need to be supported and understood. When a whole system practises defensive medicine, it is also a mirror of the lack of accountability. On a personal level, we are all responsible and accountable for our actions. How much does the NHS spend on litigious settlements? An article in The Telegraph in February 2015[*] stated that the NHS set aside a quarter of its budget for medical negligence claims. This is astounding. I was absolutely shocked to read that. How much we have all come to distrust each other at such massive cost – this computes to £26.1 billion. Imagine how funds would be better allocated if we harnessed instead a culture of trust and fair accountability. What on earth have we been doing?

I have also noted that different hospitals run different protocols. There should be, in my view, a gold standard. However, it is seemingly at the whim or discretion of the lead clinical director of the unit to determine drug protocols and the like. I know this as my friend, who attends a different hospital, is on a different drug protocol for her kidney transplant. If these differences exist locally within UK hospitals, imagine the difference in other countries. I heard that, in Japan, the donor kidney is bathed in green tea prior to transplantation. This is where cultural influence really shows up. Japan loves green tea and so the kidney gets a green tea bath! I absolutely love that. In Spain (I heard this from a Spanish nephrologist), the wait time for a kidney donor is one of the shortest in Europe. They said this was due to the Spanish being very family orientated – so if a member of the family is ill, everyone rallies round and there will be plenty of people to offer their kidney.

What support do doctors receive for their wellbeing? The NHS statistics are alarming in terms of obesity, depression and suicidal thoughts amongst

[*]by Gregory Walton, 9th February 2015, The Telegraph

its own staff. In the corporate sector, there's now a big drive for wellbeing awareness and support - we need to see this happen in our health service, too. Are we playing catch up within the health service at great cost to all involved – doctors and patients?

Meeting a doctor for the first time is effectively an exchange with a stranger. For you and for them. How often is the exchange positive and sees us come away with a sense of uplift and hope? If the chemistry is off between the two of you and the matter in hand is serious, this can have disastrous consequences.

The healer, the patient, and the environment are all key to getting well. Feeling safe is of the utmost importance and needs to be considered, by all involved. It is certainly not the case that it is just down to the physician to be the nice person. It is also for the patient to show up, be informed and take responsibility, as well as for the surrounding setting to be as pleasant as possible.

Equally, what pressure do we put on our doctors by not taking responsibility? There has to be a dialogue. Dare we ask our doctors what they would do in our situation? How can we collectively drive meaningful and positive change and transform healthcare in our society? What is your medicine? What do we understand medicine to be? To me, medicine means something that helps us towards healing. So it is not always a pill, or indeed, a supplement. It could be a hug from a loved one, it might be looking at the stars on a clear night and feeling what it is to be alive, or it might be a gin and tonic at sunset with a dear friend. Let your medicine be felt in your tissues. Also, if you are taking pharmaceuticals, bless those pills and believe they are doing you good. If you resentfully take medication, it's more likely to make you feel unwell, because you don't believe in it – and the body reacts to that.

It takes a considerable amount of energy to defend your choices to a medical professional who has not had the opportunity to explore all options, or has disconnected from their own heart and is linear, or fixed, in their views. This can present as a doctor emanating an energy of: 'I know best, don't challenge me.' Never as a doctor underestimate the knowledge and understanding of your patient. Dare you open yourself up to an open dialogue and a willing ear?

I feel that, really, this is inherently natural in all of us. We all want to connect and listen to each other at heart, but the system does not always foster that approach. The more pressure people are under, the less they are able to relax and speak from their hearts. This goes for both doctor and patient. Both are absolutely responsible for a healthy therapeutic rapport.

One appointment at the transplant clinic came at a great physical and emotional cost to me. It was during the time the kidney was still going, but only at about sixteen per cent function. I'd had a dream the night before my appointment that I was driving a car; I lost control of it and it plunged into a swimming pool. Large volumes of water in dreams can represent feeling emotionally flooded. Literally drowning in your emotions. It also represents a feeling of being out of control and unsafe, even though, symbolically, I was in the driving seat. So, when my name was called by a doctor I didn't particularly get along with, my heart sank. I just knew it was not going to go well. The unsettling dream reflected an inner knowing of what was to come. Unusually, this doctor had a very young-looking student observing. Given the context, in hindsight I should have asked for the student to leave, but I agreed she could stay. Mistake number one: I didn't listen to my instinct and speak up. These exchanges are very sensitive when things are not going well – more so when the doctor and patient have very converging views on health and life. My first issue was she had never correctly pronounced my name. I found this unprofessional after several visits. Just call me Miss Roberts if Ciara is too much! At this appointment, she went on to raise the matter of having a Hepatitis B vaccination. I stated I did not wish to have this as my body was already under great strain, and I certainly was not keen to put anything else synthetic into it. She was visibly annoyed at this, and took it as an opportunity to speak to me in a very condescending tone, made worse by the fact she had a third party to witness her bravado. It was as if she could now perform to an audience in a manner I had not previously experienced with her. I wonder if she would have been quite so bold without that audience. I felt the intensity of her tone, and it took great effort on my part to not become hysterical and shout, "Who are you to speak to me in this way?" She was basically inferring that, in order to be considered for the transplant list, they would need to know I was going to take the medications. She asked if I knew there were a lot of drugs to take at the point of surgery (um, yes I've been through it all, thanks very much), and was I going to turn up for my appointments? I was incredulous, given how I had always conducted myself. I kept saying to myself, '*Stay in your heart, stay in your heart.*' As she was talking, I started to realise she was essentially implying she wasn't going to consider listing me on the tranplant pool unless I played ball. I was horrified at the connotation, especially as no other doctor had indicated this tone to me. It absolutely was personal. I had to remain calm in order to get my point across. Any patient is completely within their rights to refuse treatment. Instinctively, I knew I did not want or need the vaccination and had not anticipated such a personal attack, which was utterly uncalled for. However, I managed to dig deep and say to her, "Yes, I know what is required." And I went on to explain that I made my decisions based on intuition, looked after myself very well, and that we all just want to be heard and understood. Whilst I had avoided becoming hysterical, I was still internally very stressed, and am sure my voice would have shown that. I was also making reference to how most of the people in the waiting room did not look very well and that the whole system was pretty broken. I was relieved when the appointment was over and she said she would document the discussion in a letter. I wondered how that would look. The whole exchange left me extremely stressed; it sank deep into my tissues, because I hadn't allowed an explosion to occur.

I then headed off to meet my sister at a spin class later that morning, and as I was feeling so impacted by that meeting, I really went for it on the spin bike. I kept up with the young males in the class, and powered the upset out of my system. This was too much. And not what my body and mind needed. It needed a comforting conversation with someone kind and understanding and for me to just breathe it out, rest it out, lift it off my body. Not long after that, I began to get itches on my skin. This turned into an insane itching that would considerably worsen at night and nearly drove me mad over the coming days. The combination of this very charged exchange with the doctor and the intense exercise that followed after had triggered eczema (much later diagnosed as that by a dermatologist, as I initially thought I had hives).

So that appointment had really cost me. My eosinophils were raised and indicated a systemic reaction. I feel for people who suffer long term with eczema. I had never experienced itching like it, and it does make you feel like you might go insane at times. Interestingly, when I travelled to Peru a few days into my yoga training, it totally went away. As soon as I was on the plane back home to London, it started to come back. It did ease again and went away fully when I got the flu, and that whole hospital episode in 2016 happened. There were many other things I did to help it, but I do find it interesting that it came along when it did. It felt like such a physically outraged response to that appointment, because it just had to come out somehow.

This is why it is so important to be understood and for doctors to open their minds to conversations with their patients. I later discovered this doctor has written papers on certain immuno-suppression drugs, which indicated to me that she was aligned very much with a 'drugs' approach.

She had not checked herself sufficiently to be able to have the awareness at the time that her behaviour was deeply inappropriate and harmful. The good news is I did see her again, and she did ask what had triggered the itching. I said, well, it was our conversation. She then paused and said, "I'm sorry." It was enough of an acknowledgement for me. By then I had processed a lot more, having been in Peru for a month with all its adventure and introspection, to know it was best to release this experience and be glad of its wisdom.

So we reconciled. I also said it was for me to respond better in such situations, and that there were no hard feelings, which I meant. In fairness, too, the letter she sent to document our appointment did state I was not keen to have the Hepatitis B vaccination as I felt it was too much for my body, and in keeping with the more natural approach I take to my health. She did also say in the appointment, after we had both ridden this intense wave, that, "we need to get our heads round how you manage your health." She went on to say she hoped I would get another kidney that would last another 20 years. So when we give ourselves time to reflect upon these challenging exchanges, we can learn from it. This goes for both the doctor and the patient. I therefore was not a victim in this exchange; I participated in it and explored its fuller meaning, in order to catalyse true change for myself. It wasn't easy, as facing yourself truthfully is often very difficult.

This same doctor was also guiding me through the mark up process for the second kidney transplant. Another requirement is to have an array of various heart tests to ensure healthy cardiovascular function ahead of such surgery. She explained to me that my heart would need to be stressed to see how it responded. To do this, I would be given an injection to create this heart stress, and that she would arrange an appointment for this. This, to me – especially after the vasopressin episode – sounded awful. And so I expressed my concern, and she agreed it might be wise to consider other options, given my sensitivity.

She proceeded to tell me that the other option was to physically challenge my heart through an exercise test. Yes! That sounds great, I'll do that, I thought. Again, if I had not questioned this, I would have been off to have that injection. Although my kidney function was very low by this point, I was still active and perfectly capable of performing what's called a CPET – a cardio-pulmonary exercise test. I actually enjoyed it when the appointment came through a few weeks later. Hooked up to a heart monitor and onto an exercise bike to power through, with two delightful cardio nurses cheering me on. And I passed with flying colours. Go, body!

I also now know much more about the dream state and how much we can learn from our dreams, which are as meaningful as our waking state. I have found, increasingly, that I can experience something in my dreams, and then when it happens, I have already processed the experience so can manage the situation much more easily. I also navigate hospital appointments in a much calmer state, as I take responsibility myself for getting so upset. Life is all about how you perceive it. And how you perceive life is influenced by so much.

At this time I was still upset, because I felt like my lovely previous doctor, the one who had been so present for me when things were starting to go off with Kenny kidney, had been stopped from seeing me. One time I did see her in the waiting room, we had a little chat and she asked me of my recent appointment, "Did they tell you to behave?" to which I replied, "No." Over the coming days, I reflected why she had asked me that, and who were 'they' she referred to. I realised that as I had stopped one of the three immuno-suppressive drugs of my own accord, because I felt it was making me sick, this would have been talked about at their wider management meetings. I could see the reaction in my mind's eye. This went some way towards explaining why this subsequent charged conversation had happened with the other doctor. Within the medical community, as in any profession, there are polarised opinions and beliefs. I know that my previous doctor was very interested in the tolerance studies and hence asked me to contribute to them, which took me on a fascinating learning curve. I know other doctors, who perhaps are more skeptical of the tolerance studies, would have seen this as her affirming my decision to cease the drugs. I had done that because I felt safe to do so and, yes, I'm sure learning about tolerance did have a bearing on my choice, because a seed of possibility had been planted. I still, however, take full responsibility for all my choices, because I know there is always a bigger picture.

The body is so complex. Consider the plethora of medical diagnoses that exist. But what is the deeper meaning of all these symptoms and physical manifestations? The current system is so fixed on the 'What' that we have lost the ability to bring the questions of 'Why' and 'How' into play. I am so grateful, during those early childhood years, to have had a doctor in South Africa who was in line with my true beliefs and instincts, and, of course, having a mother who was very aligned with this approach. Professor Thompson advised good hydration with water, eating whole foods, including plenty of plants, very limited refined sugar and no more vaccinations. The latter was relevant to my case, as vaccinations can be a burden on the kidneys. Anyone with kidney issues is wise to consider this; do your own research, before deciding what feels best for you. Live vaccines are certainly a no-no for transplant patients, as there is a the risk of the immune system being triggered negatively.

The standard clinical advice for dialysis patients, and those being marked up for the transplant pool, is to have a Hepatitis B vaccination, as per my earlier reference. As with these situations – the patient is told this is required, and the patient accepts. Sometimes that works absolutely fine, but often more questions need to be asked by the patient. If something simply doesn't feel right, it must be given a voice. For me, as my body was still recovering from the 2016 hospital episode, I definitely knew I did not want any form of vaccination. I was thankful I had already raised this with the other doctor prior to losing Kenny, and was very clear that I did not want the vaccination. This had been documented in the letter and agreed between that doctor and myself. So, months later when the transplant coordinator raised this again, I was able to reiterate that this had already been discussed. The coordinator said it would have to be raised again with the other doctor, whose care I was now under. Depending on what kidney situation you are in, your care will be managed by different people, including different clinics within the same overall renal unit, such as the low clearance clinic, transplant clinic and dialysis clinic. This meant that when I did see the doctor, he'd already been given the heads up that I wanted to talk about the vaccination. He asked at the outset of the appointment: "So, do we need to talk about the vaccination?" We then had the conversation and it transpired that vaccination is only effective in about fifty per cent of the dialysis population and, as I am a home dialysis patient, I'm at an even lower risk. I also discovered that all medical students have to get this vaccine which, I must say, surprised me. However, we had a useful discussion, and my views were once again agreed and documented. I felt even more comfortable with my decision, knowing the wider level of detail. In such instances I am in awe of my instincts, and find the more you are able to trust them, the more the universe affirms your choices. We had also a broader conversation about vaccines, as he always likes to go the extra mile and provide even more interesting information. He spoke to the benefit of some vaccinations, at which point I stepped in to say that I was not taking an anti-vaccine position per se, but that I was taking a practical view for my own health.

Statingate

An experience I had with a nephrologist I had never met before was around statins (boo hiss!). This doctor did not start off well – he didn't introduce himself, or give me any context as to who he was, after stumbling out my name in the waiting room. As we sat down in the consulting room, we started talking and I mentioned I had been having a lot of muscle fatigue and pain.

He exclaimed, "Ah, that's probably because you were prescribed statins, and that is a side effect."

Oh dear. To that I firmly responded: "I am not taking statins, and have already been very clear about this."

I'd originally been recommended a statin due to an ongoing elevated cholesterol level, triggered by the severe illness in March 2016. However, I'd trusted this would settle as my body worked to heal the systemic inflammation, and I'd said words to that effect in an email response to the original recommendation from another nephrologist, to which I never had a reply.

I remember I'd been annoyed he had recommended it in a letter, and not discussed it face-to-face with me, as he was a doctor who knew I was keen to limit exposure to prescription drugs. Statins is a class of drug I am very clear is not right for me. For me, the research does not bode well for the wider population either, and they are far too readily prescribed. I know too much about the side effects, including muscle wastage. This is very bad news for the heart, which is a major specialised muscle. So, with this new doctor I had to go over this whole topic again. He agreed and went on to say that people have actually died from taking statins. He did not seem to realise the irony of still recommending them to me, someone he had never met.

I explained how I was a yoga teacher and Nutritional Therapist, so very well versed in how to take care of this without harsh drugs. Again, the context of what I do is rarely fully understood by medics, especially when they have only their own limited training which sadly, has, no meaningful grounding in nutritional medicine – let alone the somatic healing that comes from a yoga practise.

In spite of this conversation, that doctor went on once again to recommend statins in his follow up letter to me, which I was very disheartened by. In fact, I felt crushed by it, as it spoke volumes about how little my input had been listened to. I had a bit of a meltdown, as the frustration was just too much. To me, this represents defensive medicine in action. And this was in spite of a drastic drop of two points in my cholesterol level, thanks to the many things I was doing to address the issue, which is remarkable in just a matter of weeks. I find it very concerning that there is such a culture of drug pushing. And I call it that, because that's what it is. We illegalise drugs like cocaine and cannabis, yet merrily allow potent pharmaceutical chemicals to be very available and actively prescribed onto the population. We need to stand strong in what feels right for our bodies, and not be bullied or scaremongered into taking potentially damaging drugs. Particularly when I believe there are safer and more effective ways to heal the vascular system. Again, this doesn't mean no drugs ever, just be in tune with what feels right.

At the following doctor's appointment, it was again another new, young nephrologist. However, he was actually delightful and set the scene beautifully by introducing himself, shaking my hand and meeting my gaze. He explained he was covering the clinic from another unit to help out, and I warmed to him immediately. It took less than thirty seconds for him to say that, and it made a difference.

So, imagine my chagrin when during the consultation, he again mentioned the statin and how they were continuing to recommend I take it. I had to go over this for the third time, and actually said, "I do not appreciate this drug pushing." He laughed awkwardly, but sure enough the recommendation was taken off the meds list, and the follow up letter documented that I was not keen to pursue taking statins. It took a lot to get to that stage. I then had a call a few days later from one of the nurses at the hospital, saying they had spoken to the clinic head, and suggested I take some Benecol. So although Benecol is not a product I would take, it still did signal a change in mindset: they were now suggesting a food based item instead. To me, this was actually quite a breakthrough. Slowly we climb the mountain.

In my own clinical practise, my intention is to attract people who are ready to do the inner work. Those with willing ears and open hearts, so they know it's ultimately their responsibility to foster change for themselves. In this context, I am on the other side of the therapeutic rapport, and so understand it is a considerable responsibility to take a good case history, to instill trust, and to continually build my knowledge and intuition to provide the safest and most effective advice for each person.

I do fully appreciate how 'compassion fatigue' can set in. I first heard this expression seeing a Functional Medicine General Practitioner speak at the Royal College of Physicians, and it really made me understand more the pressure doctors are under. This speaker highlighted that GPs are sometimes required to see in excess of thirty patients a day. That's a huge, energetic burden. I would be exhausted seeing that many patients in one day. I would go quite mad. This kind of insight gives enormous perspective into the day-to-day challenges that some doctors face. At this same seminar, the marvellous Dr Rangan Chatterjee was the keynote speaker. He is the face of the BBC series, Doctor in the House. A key message, as part of the wider Evolution of Medicine movement, is to have a more cohesive approach within the NHS, where nutritional therapists would work alongside doctors. This again reinforces the definite need for nutrition to be fully integrated into primary care – not to do so is a great disservice to the public. There are dieticians within the NHS, but I have had very limited experience of them. My more recent experience has by no means been bad, but it involves nowhere near the level of detail that I take when I first meet a client. That may in part be because they already know I do eat sensibly and are under time constraint. They do also have access to my records, and lab results are looking at a bigger picture, but it is all very one dimensional. The one leaflet I was given when I started

PD looked like it had been typed up in the 1980s and was very basic. The dietician who came to see me on the ward spent about five minutes with me, and that was it. I know how patients would thrive with a naturopathic approach, knowing that they are cared for and being listened to, and feeling they can empower themselves with all their choices – both in terms of food and overall lifestyle, as well as understanding the medications they are taking, and if they are absolutely necessary.

I understand too that a GP or specialist working on the NHS has no choice in who they can work with – they are at the mercy of the general public, which can also be overwhelming, as we are all so different.

And excitingly, times are changing. The area of research is now so vast and has many genuinely interested medics, statisticians and researchers looking at correlations, metadata and analysis. We are using way too many old protocols within much of allopathic medicine. For example, when renal function tails off, bicarb levels in the blood can drop. The standard protocol is for the patient to take bicarb supplements, but this can actually throw off magnesium, which is hugely detrimental to a person, especially one with impaired renal function. I did try the supplements, but they made my mood very low, and I noticed a bit of fluid retention. Instead, I opted for high bicarb mineral water. This mineral water, along with its high bicarb content, comes with other synergistic minerals, so it's potentially even more beneficial. Instinctively, this felt much better for me.

All that said – and going back to the issue of statin prescription – if you are diagnosed with high blood pressue unrelated to kidneys (inevitably though there will be some connection as everything is linked), there is plenty you can do to moderate it yourself. Medication should be last resort. I don't advise taking drugs after just one isolated reading in a doctor's office. There should be further diagnostics, and blood pressure should be monitored for 24 hours to get the fuller picture. In kidney conditions this is trickier, as they are so integral to healthy blood pressure. But it is individual and not all kidney cases will require medication for blood pressure. Also, with any blood pressure reading the physician must take an accurate reading, involving uncrossed legs and ankles, no talking, and a relaxed patient. This doesn't always happen – often the nurse or doctor will talk away whilst the blood pressure cuff is on. I then get irritated internally as this is not the correct diagnostic setting, which probably doesn't help the blood pressure!

The medical profession is not always scientific, or clear thinking. We make the assumption that they are, with sometimes serious consequences.

We must be careful of what also happens too often, when one person's piece of research widens to influence the masses, without being suitably appraised or reviewed, before it goes on to directly impact Government guidelines. It's a bit like us believing that the ratings agencies had our best interests at heart, when maintaining order within the banks, in terms of assigning appropriate ratings to investments. Of course, after the 2007/8 banking crisis it emerged that the rating agencies were in cahoots with the banks and in competition with each other, and the regulators were, for the most part, quite clueless. I do also take the view that these instances need to happen, so they prompt more meaningful and helpful action going forward. Sometimes the volcano needs to erupt, so we can seriously take stock and change our ways.

We need a whole framework that gives people options and provides the opportunity for patients to ask questions of their healthcare team, and of themselves. Operating within disjointed silos is inefficient and comes at a great cost, to both the medics and the patients. Life is connectivity and flow. How can we all create and foster a system that works using the knowledge that all is connected? I certainly do not have all the answers, but I do believe that the more we each reflect upon this and adapt our actions according to our own deeper reflection, the more this serves the whole.

I know we can create a new system. I know in my heart that it is utterly possible. If my heart knows this then so does yours, because we are all connected. We all deserve a better system. One that combines the heart-centred magic of ancient wisdom, with the technical advances and wide research of modern science. One that honours an open dialogue for all along the way. We are all collectively responsible to create this shift. The tide is changing and many are already on board. Together we can do it. It is within us all to save ourselves and future generations.

Top tips for a healthy therapeutic rapport

- Always go beyond a medical diagnosis. This means you need to ask questions of your doctor and healthcare team about what is happening, and not become your medical diagnosis. It can be very easy to literally get pushed around and rushed here and there, from appointment to appointment, especially when navigating a serious health crisis. Give yourself space to slow down. Write down questions between appointments, and bring them with you so you have a reference tool. If you are feeling particularly vulnerable and confused, take a trusted, impartial friend along to your appointments.

- Be interested in understanding your lab results; when blood-work has been taken, ask to see the results. Many units now have online Patient View, which allows you to access your results and start to explore more what they mean. Remember, too, that blood-work is just a snapshot in time. The body is always changing. Be mindful that blood serum levels of magnesium don't tell us too much about true magnesium status in the tissues.

- Check in with yourself when attending an appointment. Notice where the mind starts racing away. Deepen the breaths and take a moment, whenever you need to. Do this both before and during the appointment, as necessary. It's ok to say, 'I need a moment here.'

- Consider what medications are right for you when they are suggested. Seek to understand why a medication has been prescribed, how it is working in your body, and if it agrees with you. These are your decisions. It is always your choice.

- Lay down healthy boundaries at the outset. Be aware of your state of mind and body as you enter the consulting room. Notice where you are getting triggered. I find many people really imbibe certain phrases vocalised by their doctor and become entrenched in that. Remain fluid. There is no obligation to believe everything that is said. Maintain that clarity for yourself, so you can make wise decisions and discern the important and valid information that's applicable to you.

- Cultivate the gift of self-soothing. Especially if emotions run high following an encounter or appointment with a doctor. I would absolutely give that same advice to doctors, as they also need support. More wellbeing needs to be filtering into the NHS from a place of heart, not from a place of form over substance, or simply paying lip service to what wellbeing really means. Find ways to release stress in healthy ways, rather than addictive ones.

- In terms of the health practitioners in your life, consider who you know, like and trust. How does that impact your experience?

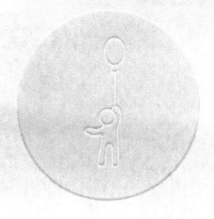

CHAPTER EIGHT

Finding joy in your recovery

As a young child, and into my teenage years, I very much wanted to heal myself. To heal my kidneys. Of course, as I've moved through my journey, I've come to know that healing comes in many forms. The unfolding is going to be what it is. And we can, indeed, heal in many ways, and this might present itself in a way we could never have imagined. This is where it is so helpful to be attentive to our experiences, so we can be aware of those moments and where shifts begin to happen. We pay attention.

For me, finding joy in my recovery has meant being fearless enough to trust my instincts. When you really allow yourself to tune into your inner environment and hear its messages and signals, your recovery becomes almost effortless. Without struggle, you feel an inner, unshakeable resilience. It is this that lead me to effectively change my whole life. To recognise I had more to offer, and to follow those instincts enough to formulate a plan and execute it. And that is how Wholly Aligned was born.

Setting up Wholly Aligned in 2013 marked a purposeful endeavour that was very much part of my own healing process. From recovery to discovery, you might say. To hold safe space for others, we need to turn inwards and dance with our own wholeness first. We then share from a place that is our natural state, rather than from a place of resentment or lack – that pervasive 'not enough' that we are all, at times, prone to. This sits in finding joy in my recovery, in that it fitted much more with who I was. We make something and then we become it. I set up Wholly Aligned, and realise now that this helped me become more in alignment with the truth of my own desires and visions.

Let me share with you how I came upon the name Wholly Aligned. I embarked on a Theta Healing course, which taps into where you are holding blocks and what your 'bottom belief' is, under certain behaviours. During this course, the word that kept coming to me was 'alignment'. Seemingly random, but this is where the more we listen to our inner voice and intuition, the more life makes sense. I was then visiting my dear long-time friend Cheryl, in the Forest of Dean, and we were sitting chatting on her outdoor trampoline on a summer's evening, with a glass of wine. We came upon the topic of words we liked, and both agreed that 'wholesome' conjured up goodness within us, and felt good to say. I went on to say how 'alignment' had been popping up a lot, and then said out loud, 'wholesome alignment' which, once vocalised, morphed into Wholly Aligned. As soon as I said it, I knew that was it. Yes!

Through experience, I have also come to feel that we truly heal by service to others. Not by neglecting our own needs and being a people pleaser, but from a heartfelt wish to help another realise their own wholeness. I very much felt this in the years Kenny kidney was easing off in function. Focusing on teaching a yoga class, or a one-to-one, I would notice afterwards I had quite forgotten my own turbulence, 'my pain'. Facilitating a class, be it a group or a private session, was uplifting. It literally lifted me out of my own junk. That is so liberating.

When I turned fifteen, I remember saying to Parley, "Will you teach me how to play the guitar?". He showed me some basic chord structures, guided me on the importance of timing, and said the rest was up to me. Isn't this so true of life? We can begin to learn what the basics are, but all the other things - what we choose to tune, refine, perfect and appreciate – are for us to determine. How will we play our unique song of life, through the wise instrument of our body? I was about one year into haemodialysis when I began to learn the guitar, and it was a beautiful and nurturing focus for me to have. I appreciated the creativity of it and enjoyed writing songs, too. This has remained a valuable companion to me over the years, and it is revealing that when I connect more with music, I feel better. Never underestimate how much your own creative expression can heal you and flood you with that quiet joy.

Part of the ongoing joy in my recovery was not being defined by my health experiences. One benefit of this coming along so early in my life was it allowed me to observe, through quite unfiltered eyes. When I saw very ill patients, I knew that was their journey. It did not need to be mine. I always had this strong sense of trust. Whilst the dialysis sessions were, at times, difficult, traumatic and took up a lot of time, I could always quite easily leave that aside as soon as the treatments were over. This really means that I was just Ciara, a teenage girl growing up in the world and exploring what it is to be human. Great joy and gratitude comes through reflection, and contemplation from a place of openness. I can look back upon those years through the lens of experience and humility. What an adventurous road I have travelled. And the journey just keeps getting better! And that is very much because I believe it to be so. This is what you might call dwelling in all possibilities. When we dwell in infinite possibilities, we are not falling into the traps of limitation.

In 2016, I was asked by the renal unit to become a Peer Supporter at the hospital. This was a meaningful marker for me. It affirmed that I was recognised as someone who had navigated my experiences, and I could share positive stories with fellow patients. I know first-hand how valuable it is to be able to talk to someone who has gone through the same experiences. I had my friend Vivien, for example: given our similar experiences, we had naturally gravitated toward one another to become firm friends, as we still are to this day. It seems only fair that I now give back as an official peer volunteer and patient representative, to help others navigate where they are, especially given my range of experience.

I remember meeting Vivien for lunch many years ago, when we were both in our 20s. She shared the news with me that she was pregnant, which was unexpected but so very joyful. I had met Vivien when we were both going for in-unit hospital haemodialysis, when at different London universities. She received her cadaveric transplant a couple of years before I did. I was very moved by this news of her pregnancy, as having a baby with a kidney transplant is considered high risk, although is more commonplace now. I shared the news with her of my engagement to my then boyfriend. Peer to peer, we met each other. Supported each other in understanding. We cried, we hoped. That is the value of meaningful mirrors in our lives. What mirrors are you dancing with at the moment? Do they reveal the darkness or the light? Both are valuable teachers. The wise tree uses both for its growth: the light from the sun to photosynthesise and the darkness of the loamy soil for nutrients into its roots. From this darkness we sprout towards the light, which helps us become lighter and to feel that in our very being.

Your capacity to heal is a blend of responsibility, understanding, surrender and belief. Facing your fears. Watching them like a movie reel in a place of safety and rest, so you don't re-trigger trauma. Instead, you get to witness it so it can be healed. Creating a safe environment to allow fears to surface; and then off they roll into the ether to be transmuted, released.

There are a few things that have stayed with me from the ten-day vipassana meditation experience and what S.N Goenka, the original Indian/Burmese teacher of vipassana, said. Firstly, there is craving and secondly, there is aversion. As humans we constantly oscillate between these two states. We crave being with someone intimately and then when we are, we are unhappy and find fault with the other. We are then in aversion to them. We crave a better job and then when we do find one, we feel too much pressure. In this type of cycle it becomes very challenging to experience happiness. We have become enslaved by our survivalist minds. And so, we look towards cultivating equanimity. A balanced state of being, so our hearts can soar. This, however, takes ongoing commitment.

Part of the recovery process is also found in the support of friends and family, and the golden nuggets that come forth every now and then, when we are open to hearing them. When I was much younger, not long after I had started haemodialysis, I recall being in the kitchen of our family home in Dorset. I was quite upset and stropping around a bit, in a very teenage way, about my situation – probably to do with having messed up the cooking of the potatoes, which needed to be double boiled to release as much potassium out of them as possible. I over-cooked them, and they looked so pitiful and representative of the mush that I was feeling, I just had a surge of anger pulse through me at the darkness.

Parley said to me, "Ciara, there is always someone else worse off than you." He said it in a very calm way and I remember it landed very much with me. Life is contextual. Sometimes, we need to be reminded of our good fortune and all the many positives there are. It was a valuable moment for me, as it gave me the gift of understanding perspective and to cease a potent negative inner dialogue with myself. That perspective breaks up the density of negative thoughts. Laughter also does this, which is why it's so important to roar with belly laughter as much as possible. The brain, by nature, is constantly on alert for risk. This is a safeguard for us, but we mustn't view everything as potential risk. We have created a world on this basis, particularly in the West.

I remember clearly a conversation with my best friend Anna, when she had come to visit at a time when I wasn't feeling great, and there were so many question marks over what was happening with Kenny kidney. I was exhausted and depleted on all levels. She simply said, "Give your body the right message." It helped me hugely to hear that. So simple and so relevant: to let the mind sabotaging settle and the internal dialogue become more hopeful.

An extremely joyful part in my recovery, following the transplant in 1997, was going travelling with my friend Jenny the following year. It started off with Jenny asking me if I wanted to go to South Africa with her for a few months. We were both born there so it seemed a natural fit to return together. However, based on my instincts, I instead suggested we go somewhere neither of us had been and have a real working experience in that place. So off we went. We started off with a month of fun and general raucousness in Australia, followed by six months in New Zealand. After this we visited Fiji, Raratonga, had a fleeting few days in Hawaii, and completed our travels in the USA. We visited California first, where we connected with my aunt and cousin, and then went up to Vancouver Island before a final stop in New York. We met so many lovely people along the way, and had such fun and, as Parley said, it was my rite of passage. I travelled on my own terms and was responsible for myself. It was only more recently, at Jenny's dear father's funeral that Parley said to Jenny, "That was a big thing you did, heading off with Ciara so soon after her transplant." I had never looked at it that way but, all those years later, it made me see things from another perspective. It was probably a worrying time for my parents, seeing me off for nine months around the world after the whirlwind years of dialysis and transplantation. But I also realised it was a dear thing for our friendship that Jenny and I both trusted each other to do it, and that neither of us made a big deal or an issue about it – we were just two young beans off for big adventures, and that was that!

Soon after we arrived in Auckland after our hectic month in Oz, we became two sloths and lazed about in a central hostel for about ten days. The most strenuous thing we did was get up and have coffee and muffins and slowly consider our work options (as we had come to Auckland on working visas, so wanted to find work). During that time I got a chest infection. It was still just over one-year post transplant, when any infection was worrying, so it was best to get it checked out. So off we went to Auckland Hospital, and the staff there could not have been lovelier. The hospital in Oxford had given me details of who to get in touch with so I could be under a doctor's care whilst away. And I was not charged a penny. What a kindness. As I needed a chest x-ray, I was attired in the attractive open backed gowns, perhaps appropriate for show-casing butt dancing. I remember Jenny laughing, saying I looked like Mr Burns from The Simpsons. There was no cause for concern. A chest infection was diagnosed and it cleared up fine with a course of antibiotics. I was at the time only 22 and did not have the wealth of experience I now have around antibiotics, and how to support yourself after a course. The naiveté a gift of youth, one might say. During the nine months of our travels, there were no other health concerns that were not manageable. At one appointment, I remember the doctor taking my blood pressure and it was pretty elevated. He was frank with me, and said it needed to be under control otherwise I'd be dead by 50. Whilst this did shock me – I called Jenny straight after the appointment in tears, and she came home from work to comfort me – I can see that kind of frank advice is, at times, appropriate. And he did not relay it in a controlling or unkind way, he just made a statement that made sense, as he was an older, experienced physician looking at a 22 year-old young woman. As a result of that I took better care of myself, eased off the alcohol and went to see a Chinese Medicine practitioner who gave me some tea and herbs. This brought it back to a much healthier level, along with allopathic blood pressure medication. It had not entered my mind that there would be health issues whilst we were travelling around the world, so these Auckland Hospital events did not really unsettle me. I just had an innate confidence in my recovery and how I was – although some days I did feel rubbish and exhausted. When that happened, I would rest. And then be delighted when I felt improved. Jenny was also a very grounded friend and never panicked. This was perfect, as the last thing I get on with is drama and panic – especially when it comes to my own health.

In 2013 when my kidney took a turn, it was an exhausting time. Firstly the knock-on physiological impact of the kidney beginning to go offline, in terms of energy and general malaise. Secondly, of course, the emotional rollercoaster and not knowing what's coming next – particularly after having had a smooth run for so many years. Was it curtains for Kenny? Will things stabilise? At what levels will they stabilise – and will that be enough to keep me feeling well? I was still working in private banking at this time and my line manager was so kind. She could see my health concerns were genuine and that my fatigue was very out of character for someone who usually takes on her work with gusto, and multi-tasks with great efficiency – including roaring at badly behaved bankers! I was pleased to be open enough to keep her in the loop with what was going on and why I needed to go for regular hospital appointments. I worked from home when necessary, to take some pressure off myself. One week was particularly tough. I was emotionally exhausted from being at the forefront of having to face my fears. And being someone usually very active and involved with both work and a social life, I could feel things were just totally out of flow. It was my old school friend Cheryl who said to me, "You need to just rest and the most strenuous thing you should do is make yourself a green tea. Just take everything right down." This was timely and wonderful advice. And so, I told my boss I was taking a week off to rest and process everything. I did not want to run and hide from this. Of course, it's not easy when you're in the storm. But I knew it was a crucial part of my healing. I had to look my fears straight in the face, address them, feel them and explore them. I had to shine the light on them to dissipate their hold. This is 'The Great Work,' as my wonderful shamanic teacher, Don Oscar Miro Quesada, says. And I understand why it is called that. It is a gift to do this work and to dance with your darkness to discover who you really are.

Who are you beneath the cloaks of stories, and how much energy are you expending keeping old stories alive?

Share your story, heal your soul. This was a strap-line in an American magazine that I cut out and made it part of a vision board I crafted with my cousin Lisa, in January 2016. It was part of a vision we were both creating for ourselves as we tucked ourselves up into the beautiful Briar Patch Inn in Sedona, Arizona, which is one of my favourite sanctuaries.

Surrounded by the imposing mineral rich, red rock that is characteristic of Sedona, we both made a vision board each, and shared our hopes and dreams with each other as part of a new year ritual. We soaked our feet in epsom salts, did face masks and were in bed before midnight. A soothing start to 2016 – a year that would bring great possibilities to transform. That strap line has stayed with me ever since, and I have come to understand its meaning more truthfully. It was an important point in time to plant this seed of sharing, of speaking more freely, of losing the potent charge of painful memory. It helped me to almost effortlessly step into the fortitude of sharing my experiences.

One day in Spring 2018, whilst sitting in the renal outpatients' department, ahead of a standard two monthly nurse review, I looked around to see several poster size pictures of me, standing in tree pose, on the walls within the unit. I was slightly taken aback, as I thought they would be on display just for one day when I'd come along to help out months ago, as part of a dialysis roadshow. The posters still remain up for all to see. This photograph had been taken by my sister in her garden in Summer 2017, after I was asked by one of the nurses to share my story and provide a picture of me doing yoga, with the catheter showing. It was to demonstrate that life goes on and remains full of hope and possibility, of movement and joy. Who would have thought I could be a yogic poster girl for wellness in the hospital! Before everything of the past few years happened, I just wanted to go to my appointments, keep them brief and skip out again. And now there I am, fully exposed and glad to share. The picture revealed the abdominal catheter, albeit covered with the usual dressings. I just had on a pair of leggings and a crop top. That, for me, represents a huge shift. It also means that the potent charge of past years has very much dissipated. I don't need to view my life through the lens of limitation or great sadness. It is possible to live moment to moment, in the richness of the present, so to be free from the stories of our past. That is liberation. However, this work never ends. Every day is a commitment to stay present and not get lost in the stories.

About a week after I came out of hospital in 2016, my sister and her two children came to visit. I wanted to be very open with my niece and nephew, who were seven and nine at the time, so I said to the little people, "Now, I just need to let you know I have a tube in my belly and that I have a machine that is helping keep me well, as my kidney alone is not able to do that." I had said this as my niece, the younger of the two and a very self-aware little thing, looked me square in the eyes as she always does, and said, "Now, are you better?" She still asks me now and then, "Do you still have your tube? When is it coming out?" She also makes reference from time to time about how we all had flu at the same time, but wasn't it curious that it had made me so sick. I have reassured her that me getting the flu from them was just one of those things and it was absolutely not their fault. You never know how a child might interpret something or begin to take responsibility for something. It makes life much easier when we just say what is going on and are more open. This has definitely been a process for me, and the more I have stepped into the joy of living from my heart, the more open I am about telling people what's going on, without a care in the world. In previous years, that kind of openness might have been very challenging for me. I felt the potency and charge of repressed emotion too much.

This very openness showed up one Saturday morning in the Crystal Palace food market, when I happened upon one of its co-founders, who is a lovely and very knowledgeable woman. I was feeling very comfortable within myself and as we chatted, I started to tell her about my health situation. Little did I know that this would plant a seed and see her invite me to share my personal story at a series of food and health talks she was arranging with a former nephrologist. I agreed. I was ready to step into my power to speak openly and inspirationally about the sojourn. I absolutely loved the talk and had wonderful feedback. This set me on a path of stating that I was ready to walk in the shoes of an inspirational speaker. And of course, once I did that, more doors opened. Rather than terrifying me, this sharing lit a fire in my belly. I know the fire I have walked through has brought me to this joyful space, of communicating through the power of an uplifting and hopeful story.

A few years ago I attended a weekend of talks, as part of the London *I Can Do It* hosted by Hay House, a large publishing house set up by the metaphysician, Louise Hay. There was plenty of inspiration from all the wonderful speakers. I do recall one specific quote from a Mexican father and son team who spoke together. The father was don Miguel Ruiz, and he'd had a heart transplant. He made the statement: "Deeply inquire in order to deeply respond" and I felt it strongly resonate. Yes, in order to experience joy through the transcendence of our suffering, we must deeply inquire of ourselves and allow ourselves to be with the responses that arise. This is where a practise such as yoga is so useful. It provides the space and stillness to look within. As one of my private yoga clients said to me, "There aren't many opportunities in life to be in a safe space to feel our feelings." Why have we created such an over-excited state of existence? We must calm our brains and listen more to the song of our heart. When we do move towards stillness, the answers will surface from within. No true solution is outside of yourself. It always comes from within. When I started to have the experience of losing Kenny's function, I reached inwards in order to then reach out. I trusted I would find solutions. I came across the naturopathic doctor, Dr Jenna Henderson, whilst browsing on an online kidney transplant forum. I contacted her and we arranged a Skype appointment where she gave me practical and safe tips, in terms of food and supplements, along with the advice to belly laugh daily! Such powerful medicine, with only blissful side effects. Interestingly, she was not only a naturopathic doctor with a wealth of knowledge based on well researched, evidence-based advice, she has also been through the experience of dialysis and transplantation. I found taking this type of practical action from a safe source very reassuring, and took on board all the advice she gave. I'm sure at the time this helped my body to stabilise. It was around this time that, although the kidney had been badly impacted and declined, this suddenly ceased and hung in there at about seventeen per cent. Enough to be enough for now. Around the same time, my dear friend Dana recommended I get in touch with an energy healer she knew. And this began a very meaningful few years of working with him. At times this was not easy, as he did pose certain questions of me; of my deeper existence and patterns. I had to keep looking into the pool of memories and to see what I was still holding onto, and how I really felt about myself.

Around this time I took the decision to step away completely from the corporate world, and everything started to open up. For example, I connected more with my neighbours, who before I don't even remember seeing, even though we'd all lived in the same place for a number of years. This change in pace and inner work allowed me to forge more connections with a happier and much more peaceful life. I could see my parents more regularly, and Marley would often come to London in the week and we would go for coffee, chats and lunch, or sometimes a glass of wine. These are such rich experiences to nourish the heart. I also began doing 'swaps' with other practitioners, who would often then become very good friends. I still do a number of these now and it's a very special way to work with people. One treatment swapped for another. For example, I regularly see an osteopath and, in exchange, I see her for a nutrition or yoga session. This, to me, represents sacred reciprocity. Money does not feature in these particular type of exchanges – the value comes from the treatment and the intention behind the treatment, to truly help one another. This then helps one's recovery become an adventure. Forget throwing yourself off a mountain or whitewater rafting –adventure can be felt in these types of navigations, so we come to truly understand who we are, why we are and where we are meant to be going. A health crisis can be an adventure if you choose to view it in that way. When my kidney was going offline, I remember saying to my friend Vivien that I was going to look at the next kidney transplant as a project, and be really excited about it. Now, that doesn't mean it was excitement all the way. It required showing up for myself – and, at times, some very uncomfortable conversations. Once the inner compass has been located, the path became clearer. It's not without obstacle, but less obstructed by the mind's limited view, and experienced more from the wisdom and compassion of the heart. Your heart yearns to connect with you.

Consider, too, who your role models and true supporters are on your journey. Who are the people who are truly those who provide sustenance to you, through the warmth they radiate? When I was in my teens, I remember us as a family watching, with great joy and almost disbelief, the brilliant Jonah Lomu, the superstar rugby player for the New Zealand All Blacks. Not only did he have tremendous skill as a rugby player, he moved like a bullet, with the pure power of speed and agility. He was also in my mind when I travelled to New Zealand. I later learned that he had kidney issues and eventually required a kidney transplant. I admired his strength and figured, if he could play world class rugby with his kidney condition, then anything was possible. I was heartbroken and wept when I read he'd died, at only 40 years old, having been back on dialysis for a number of years. It felt at that time that all dreams can be shattered. I realised I needed to forge ahead and continue to be my own role model, as well as for others. I must show myself what is possible, so this shines a light for others.

And inspiration will always come. I was watching the London world athletics in summer 2017 and was thrilled to hear about Aries Merritt, an American 110m hurdler and event world record holder, whose sister gifted him a kidney. He had been competing at a world class level without realising he had focal segmental glomerulosclerosis, which was what necessitated this kidney donation in 2015. It is tremendous that he has continued to live his dream and come back strong and healthy. There he was, just two years later, competing at such a standard. This gives such a positive message. I know what strength this will have taken on his part.

Keep an open mind to synchronicity in your life. When I came out of hospital in 2016, I was delighted when the latest online *Deepak and Oprah 21 Day Meditation* was announced. Deepak Chopra is a well known leader and author in the field of spirituality. Oprah is probably the most famous talk show host in the world - so for them to have come together and collaborated on these regular, free meditations is just wonderful. They always have a particular theme and are only about 20 minutes a day, and include an introduction from Oprah followed by a mantra and meditation by Deepak. And guess what the theme was at that time? Finding joy in your recovery. That is synchronicity, as it reflected so deeply what I was feeling. There were many other instances of this, all there to connect the dots when we are open to doing so. Another example was when, in 2015, I treated myself to custom built floor-to-ceiling wardrobes in my bedroom. This turned out to be not only a great addition to my flat, but very handy when I needed to commence home dialysis, as there are significant amounts of medical supplies needed. This includes fluid bags, the extension lines to drain, the cassettes to attach to the machine so things flow in and out where they should, and all the ancillary bits and pieces, such as gauze dressings and sterilising wipes. I'd also done that big Mari Kondo clear out at the beginning of 2016, so my wardrobes were actually quite sparse and, as a result, there was good space for storage of the medical supplies, which was very fortunate. The first delivery I had was an overwhelming moment for me and I did have a little cry. There were seventy boxes and I wondered how on earth I was going to store it all. The last thing you want is to feel like your home has become a clinic. But, thanks to the storage space in my clear wardrobes, it worked out. It was as if my flat just adapted and took care of it.

I'm also continually overjoyed with the way in which the world supports me to live as easily as possible, considering the challenges this equipment and treatment could bring. I feel supported because I believe I am supported. Therefore, this becomes my experience.

The local council deliver clinical waste bags and come once a week to collect the used equipment. I get monthly deliveries of the medical supplies. There are several components, therefore, to this all running smoothly, and I am thankful for all the cogs in the wheel. If the council men come in their big waste disposal truck when I am in, I waft waves of gratitude their way for their weekly efficiency. I have also found travelling abroad to be enlightening, in terms of the ease with which the airline crew accept I am travelling with a dialysis machine. The machine, along with its case, checks in at about 25kg, and needs to go in the hold. They tag it and direct me to the airport's special items section. They know it is free of charge as it is life supporting medical equipment, so there is never any quibble around excess baggage charges. It all just works.

I also embraced self-care on a profound level. I recommend self-care to my clients and remain attentive to this for myself. So I'll have a massage and regular reflexology, as well as taking time to just be. I spend time with my favourite uplifting people and take rest when needed. I am kind to myself in practical and spiritual ways. To me, coming home with a PD machine was a step that was very much in line with the importance of self-care. It turned out to be such an extraordinarily positive and different experience to those years of in-unit hospital haemodialysis. In time, I managed to set up the machine in little over ten minutes. It's recommended you set it up earlier in the day because, come bedtime, you will feel tired, and more likely to make a mistake. So I usually do that in the late afternoon, which my current lifestyle allows, and then can just plug in and hop into bed later for the eight hour treatment. With the residual function of my donor kidney preserved, passing urine is wonderful, so there is no fluid restriction and no real restrictions diet wise, because my blood chemistry remains pretty good. Obviously that is in the context of me being a nutritionist and very well versed in how to look after myself.

I have one night a week off, which means my current regime is eight hours nightly, six nights a week. If I am going away for a weekend, I do take two nights off and that's mostly fine. On some occasions I do feel ready for dialysis by the time two nights and three days have passed. I might do this every couple of months. I did take two nights off when I was sick with the flu to prioritise sleep and rest, and that was also fine. In fact, infection risk increases with any virus or cold, so it is better to skip dialysis until the infection has passed.

I am also very cognisant that dialysis is quite environmentally burdensome. It's imperative to follow the aseptic technique, which means thorough hand washing when I am setting up the machine or changing my catheter dressing, but this means running the water for up to two minutes each time. Each nightly treatment also generates a fair amount of plastic waste, as there are four separate fluid bags, plus the drain lines and cassettes. I make up for this by mostly strip washing. Baths are not allowed due to infection risk so at least it evens out, and I save water that way. Showers are fine, so I also balance out water usage by not showering every day.

When you open doors for yourself, you open doors for others and allow yourself to be seen more clearly. One of the joyful experiences I had from my 2016 awakening was to more fully and completely follow my instincts. One of these was to write to the main surgeon at my kidney transplant in October 1997 – the one I'd given the Tigger to. I managed to find where he was using the internet, and discovered he was now based in Cambridge. He had actually only been in Oxford for one year – so I was so lucky to have had him there for my surgery. I wanted to express my thanks to him and give him an update, nearly two decades on. So I wrote him a letter that, at its heart, was one of thanks. Thanks to him for his skill as a surgeon and as a human being. It felt absolutely the right thing for me to do, and I had no expectation to hear from him, so quite forgot about it. Some weeks later, a letter arrived with a lovely letterhead from the University of Cambridge, and it was a reply from him! It was such a touching letter, and I was very moved he had taken the time to respond and acknowledge my reaching out. He said he did indeed remember me and that he still had his Tigger up on his wall clock, out of reach of the dog. This made me cry. It was such a personal image to bring to mind as I still have my Tigger, gifted by the nurses that same Christmas. He went on to frame his words with such sensitivity around the drugs situation, which I had briefly mentioned in my letter to him. He wrote: "It is frustrating that the level of tolerance you achieved is so brittle." That sums it up so well. I was heartened by his letter and so glad I trusted my instincts to write to him. He wished me well and hoped a kidney would come up soon. He also affirmed I would be well looked after by the team in London. He had trained with a couple of the surgeons that are there now, and assured me they had a great reputation. Support always comes. It really does. That letter meant so much to me.

This exchange led to me reaching out to him two years later, to talk to him about this book. He is still a busy surgeon, and I was very fortunate to go and visit him in Cambridge. It's difficult to describe fully how that felt. When I saw him for the first time in over two decades, it was almost as if time had stood still. He really hadn't changed much. I came away reflecting what did I know about anything? People are living their lives in their own contexts, and doing the best they can in their own circumstances. A big realisation, as I thought about this over the following few days, was what a gift it is to have a purpose. This surgeon clearly enjoys what he does, even though the environment he's in is often very challenging, due to a lack of staff, long hours and almost persistently being on call. As I had chatted to him about his working world, it was clear he felt there was a collegiate approach to helping each other within his team, and he absolutely had a sense of purpose – he has transformed hundreds of lives through skilful kidney, liver and pancreas transplants. That sense of purpose can drive and sustain someone so deeply and richly. He was still driven to do this, even after years of sleep deprivation and perhaps not the best exercise regime – as he has no time for that. In the yogic world, we call this dharma. And I feel that sense of purpose too, deep in my soul, and know that is what keeps me so well.

I have not always made good choices along the way. Sometimes I self-sabotaged, and there were times, when I was younger, that I did not really take such an interest in my blood results. I have not always been consistent. Give yourself time to adjust and make changes. Be open. Ask questions. Be curious. Mistakes made often turn out to be incredibly valuable lessons of what not to do and how not to behave. We not only learn from these mistakes, we are transformed by them. Learning can fade, but transformation lasts. For example, it was only after the fact that I spotted on my records I had started leaking protein, which is a strong indicator of kidney health. No-one had told me, but there's no point in saying: if I'd known then, I could have recovered, or prevented the inflammatory process that started. But this discovery was a reminder to me to pay attention to all results, and to know what diagnostics were relevant to me and how to interpret them – and, of course, apply my own clinical experience to the situation. I am then able to use this same knowledge in how I work with my own clients.

The Darwinian belief of survival of the fittest is very outdated. Any healthy functioning community, be it humans or within the animal kingdom, is only as strong as its weakest link. So how we then treat – or, indeed, embrace – the weakest link is so important. We must question, we must be courageous, and we must tune into what feels best for us. Courage is not an absence of fear, it is the resilience of overcoming the fear. The fear is still there, just not taking over.

We can accept the turbulence and that it is a part of us. We massive surge in over-medicating our feelings, or turning away through the prescription of anti-depressants. We all feel turbulenc pain and suffering, because we are all human. Over-medicating with brain-centric system creates a bigger disconnect with the wise energy o the heart. Light and dark are two sides of the same coin. We are not all skipping through life effortlessly, with a permanent smile upon our face. It's ok to feel darkness and sadness and pain. We must embrace it and find truly helpful ways to lessen its grip upon us. So we keep asking of our hearts: heart, please guide me, help me understand that I am not at the mercy of my thoughts.

It took me a long time to find my way to my heart. I knew it was always within me, but the darkness and suffering would, at times, sweep over me. I had thoughts of wanting to exit this life, which was not just related to my health situation. If we are not careful, heartbreak from the end of an intimate relationship creates such pain and closes off our connection to our hearts.

Within seconds of meeting me, a wise woman in Peru said to me: "There is a great sadness within you." I immediately began to cry. And she went on to say, "You need to learn to live more from your heart." She also told me the energy flowed very strongly within me, even though I had a kidney transplant. It affirmed to me that I am deeply fortunate to feel this inner strength. It sounds so simple to live from your heart, yet it took me some time to really understand what that meant, and to this day it continues to be a deep exploration. And I'm still learning! However, each day I now connect with gratitude. When I get into bed each night, I bring to mind three things from the day that I am grateful for. By practising gratitude in this way, you can connect more with your heart, and realise your gifts and blessings. You can retrain the mind to come away from the fixation with negative bias. It is important we understand that turbulence and suffering are part of the great wheel of life, along with joy and love. How

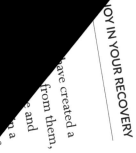

...e haven't experienced suffering? Think of
...nd still, sometimes it roars and churns
...it will never again settle. But it does. It
...dysfunctional; that is just its nature, as is
...us.

...has also been about connecting more with
...oar. That voice from deep within, suppressed for so long, has
been given a platform through this book, and all the other work I am so so
fortunate to be doing. This is, indeed, a very personal story. I have chosen
to present it based on how I feel and how I recall my experiences. It is not
an exercise in intellectual reasoning or me trying to convince you to do
this or that. I'm simply sharing my experiences. Inevitably, there are more
questions to seek answers to, as well as deeper considerations. This will
always be ongoing – and sometimes we just might not get the answers,
which is where we learn to accept and surrender. Further work on my
part will still be done. I have more to research, more to experience, more
people to speak with and be inspired by – within both the communities
of physicians and of patients. I'm interested to hear more about where
our views converge and where we might fill in the gaps for each other. As
Louise Hay says, "Change the world, start a conversation."

I'm so grateful for the life I have lived. I'm so grateful for the care I have
received, in all aspects of my health. I see now how it all formed part of my
initiation into understanding the human experience deeply. I am blessed
to live a life I truly love, and with the capacity to continue to grow and
evolve. That doesn't mean it's always easy, but when there is a grounding in
acceptance of what comes, and a willingness to grow from it, what a joyful
gift that is. We have then indeed awakened our inner physician.

Tips for finding joy in your recovery

- Practise gratitude daily. I do this at night time, when I get into bed and once the lights are out, lying down and bringing to mind three things from that day that I am grateful for. This will over time re-orientate your inner world. It is also a beautiful setting in which to allow the mist of sleep to descend.

- Smile at strangers. I am another you. Acknowledge your fellow souls walking this earth.

- Self-care with things that make you feel good. Absolutely embrace the warm and fuzzy feelings.

- Take time out to heal and don't feel guilty about it. It is so worth giving yourself that space in the long run.

- Follow your intuition. You might know it more as your gut instinct, or sixth sense. We all have it, I assure you. Interestingly, having a healthy gut will help you connect more with your intuition. Healthy gut, healthy intuitive instinct.

- Speak about how you are. Be unafraid to share. My journey has been a huge shift for me from being very private about my health, to being much more open. An example was visiting one of my favourite cafes in Crystal Palace, The Blackbird. Much of this book was birthed there – so it absolutely deserves a mention! After coming out of hospital in 2016, the lovely James in The Blackbird asked how I was, without knowing anything of my personal situation. I was feeling so open and balanced and in my body, I told him how I had been in hospital, had lost my kidney function, and was doing home dialysis. He was utterly unphased by this and went on to share how his Grandfather had renal failure, and had lasted 10 years on haemodialysis at a ripe old age.

I love that I received that story, in exchange for sharing such an equally exposing piece of information. Life goes on.

Lightning Source UK Ltd.
Milton Keynes UK
UKHW020635221221
396077UK00009B/485